Lecture Notes in Computer Science 8549

Commenced Publication in 1973
Founding and Former Series Editors:
Gerhard Goos, Juris Hartmanis, and Jan van Leeuwei

Xiaolong Zheng   Daniel Zeng
Hsinchun Chen   Yong Zhang
Chunxiao Xing Daniel B. Neill (Eds.)

Smart Health

International Conference, ICSH 2014
Beijing, China, July 10-11, 2014
Proceedings

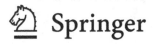

Springer

Volume Editors

Xiaolong Zheng
Chinese Academy of Sciences, Beijing, China
E-mail: xiaolong.zheng@ia.ac.cn

Daniel Zeng
The University of Arizona, Tucson, AZ, USA
and
Chinese Academy of Sciences, Beijing, China
E-mail: zeng@email.arizona.edu

Hsinchun Chen
The University of Arizona, Tucson, AZ, USA
and
Tsinghua University, Beijing, China
E-mail: hchen@eller.arizona.edu

Yong Zhang
Chunxiao Xing
Tsinghua University, Beijing, China
E-mail: {zhangyong05; xingcx}@tsinghua.edu.cn

Daniel B. Neill
Carnegie Mellon University, Pittsburgh, PA, USA
E-mail: neill@cs.cmu.edu

ISSN 0302-9743   e-ISSN 1611-3349
ISBN 978-3-319-08415-2   e-ISBN 978-3-319-08416-9
DOI 10.1007/978-3-319-08416-9
Springer Cham Heidelberg New York Dordrecht London
Library of Congress Control Number: 2014941597
LNCS Sublibrary: SL 3 – Information Systems and Application, incl. Internet/Web
and HCI

Typesetting: Camera-ready by author, data conversion by Scientific Publishing Services, Chennai, India

Printed on acid-free paper

Springer is part of Springer Science+Business Media (www.springer.com)

Preface

Advancing Informatics for healthcare and healthcare applications has become an international research priority. There is increased effort to transform reactive care to proactive and preventive care, clinic-centric to patient-centered practice, training-based interventions to globally aggregated evidence, and episodic response to continuous well-being monitoring and maintenance. The annual International Conference for Smart Health (ICSH) began in 2013. This first conference, held in Beijing, attracted over 50 contributors and participants from all over the world, providing a forum for meaningful multidisciplinary interactions.

The 2014 International Conference for Smart Health (ICSH 2014) was organized to develop a platform for authors to discuss fundamental principles, algorithms or applications of intelligent data acquisition, processing and analysis of healthcare information. Specifically, this conference mainly focused on topics and issues including information sharing, integrating and extraction, clinical practice and medical monitoring, clinical and medical data mining, and large-scale health data analysis and management. We are pleased that many high-quality technical papers were submitted, accompanied by evaluation with real world data or application contexts. The work presented at the conference encompassed a healthy mixing of computer science, medical informatics, and information systems approaches.

ICSH 2014 was held in Beijing, China. The 1.5-day event encompassed presentations of 24 papers. The organizers of ICSH 2014 would like to thank the conference sponsors for their support and sponsorship, including Tsinghua University, the Chinese Academy of Sciences, National Natural Science Foundation of China, and University of Arizona. We also greatly appreciate the following technical co-sponsors, Institute for Operations Research and the Management Sciences (INFORMS), ACM Beijing Chapter, and China Association for Information Systems. We further wish to express our sincere gratitude to all Program Committee members of ICSH 2014, who provided valuable and constructive review comments.

July 2014

Xiaolong Zheng
Daniel Zeng
Hsinchun Chen
Yong Zhang
Chunxiao Xing
Daniel B. Neill

Organizing Committee

Conference Co-chairs

Hsinchun Chen — University of Arizona, USA; Tsinghua University, China

Daniel Zeng — University of Arizona, USA; Chinese Academy of Sciences, China

Chunxiao Xing — Tsinghua University, China

Program Co-chairs

Xiaolong Zheng — Chinese Academy of Sciences, China

Yong Zhang — Tsinghua University, China

Daniel Neill — Carnegie Mellon University, USA

Tutorial Co-chairs

John Brownstein — Harvard Medical School, USA

Hsin-Min Lu — National Taiwan University, Taiwan

Zhidong Cao — Chinese Academy of Sciences, China

Finance Co-chairs

Hui Yang — University of South Florida, USA

Ahmed Abbasi — University of Virginia, USA

Donald Adjeroh — West Virginia University, USA

Poster Chair

Howard Burkom — Johns Hopkins University, USA

Yongqiang Lyu — Tsinghua University, China

Publication Co-chairs

Wendy Chapman — University of California at San Diego, USA

Scott Leischow — Mayo Clinic, USA

Chao Li — Tsinghua University, China

Publicity Co-chairs

Kwok Tsui City	University of Hong Kong, China
Guandong Xu	University of Technology, Sydney, Australia

Program Committee

Yigal Arens	University of Southern California, USA
Ian Brooks	University of Illinois at Urbana-Champaign, USA
David Buckeridge	McGill University, Canada
Nitesh V. Chawla	University of Notre Dame, USA
Guanling Chen	University of Massachusetts Lowell, USA
Kup-Sze Choi	The Hong Kong Polytechnic University, Hong Kong SAR, China
Kainan Cui	Xi'an Jiaotong University, China
Amar Das	Dartmouth College, USA
Ron Fricker	Naval Postgraduate School, USA
Hassan Ghasemzadeh	University of California at Los Angeles, USA
Natalia Grabar	STL CNRS Université Lille 3, France
Takahiro Hara	Osaka University, Japan
Saike He	Chinese Academy of Sciences, China
Xiaohua Hu	Drexel University, USA
Kun Huang	The Ohio State University, USA
Roozbeh Jafari	University of Texas at Dallas, USA
Ernesto Jimenez-Ruiz	University of Oxford, UK
Victor Jin	The Ohio State University, USA
Hung-Yu Kao	National Cheng Kung University, Taiwan
Kenneth Komatsu	Arizona Department of Health Services, USA
Erhun Kundakcioglu	University of Houston, USA
Feipei Lai	National Taiwan University, Taiwan
Gondy Leroy	Claremont Graduate University, USA
Jiao Li	Chinese Academy of Medical Sciences, China
Xiaoli Li	Institute for Infocomm Research, Singapore
Chuan Luo	Chinese Academy of Sciences, China
Mohammad Mahoor	University of Denver, USA
Jin-Cheon Na	Nanyang Technological University, Singapore
Radhakrishnan Nagarajan	University of Kentucky, USA
Balakrishnan Prabhakaran	University of Texas at Dallas, USA
Xiaoming Sheng	University of Utah, USA
Min Song	New Jersey Institute of Technology, USA
Xing Tan	University of Ottawa, Canada
Chunqiang Tang	IBM Research, USA

Cui Tao	Mayo Clinic, USA
Vincent S. Tseng	National Cheng Kung University, Taiwan
Egon L. Van Den Broek	TNO / University of Twente / Radboud UMC Nijmegen, The Netherlands
Jason Wang	New Jersey Institute of Technology, USA
May D. Wang	Georgia Institute of Technology and Emory University, USA
Chunhua Weng	Columbia University, USA
Jinglong Wu	Okayama University, Japan
Bo Xie	University of Texas at Austin, USA
Christopher Yang	Drexel University, USA
Hui Yang	University of South Florida, USA
Mi Zhang	University of Southern California, USA
Yanchun Zhang	Victoria University, Australia
Zhu Zhang	Chinese Academy of Sciences, China
Kai Zheng	The University of Michigan, USA

Table of Contents

Information Sharing, Integrating and Extraction

Health Data Analysis and Management

Clinical and Medical Data Mining

Clinical Practice and Medical Monitoring

Emoticon Analysis for Chinese Health and Fitness Topics

Shuo Yu[1], Hongyi Zhu[1], Shan Jiang[2], and Hsinchun Chen[1,2]

[1] School of Economics and Management, Tsinghua University, Beijing, China
{yush.10,zhuhy.10}@sem.tsinghua.edu.cn
[2] Department of Management Information Systems, University of Arizona, Tucson, U.S.
jiangs@email.arizona.edu, hchen@eller.arizona.edu

Abstract. An emoticon is a metacommunicative pictorial representation of facial expressions, which serves to convey information about the sender's emotional state. To complement non-verbal communication, emoticons are frequently used in Chinese online social media, especially in discussions of health and fitness topics. However, limited research has been done to effectively analyze emoticons in a Chinese context. In this study, we developed an emoticon analysis system to extract emoticons from Chinese text and classify them into one of 7 affect categories. The system is based on a kinesics model which divides emoticons into semantic areas (eyes, mouths, etc.), with an improvement for adaption in the Chinese context. Empirical tests were conducted to evaluate the effectiveness of the proposed system in extracting and classifying emoticons, based on a corpus of more than one million sentences of Chinese health- and fitness-related online messages. Results showed the system to be effective in detecting and extracting emoticons from text, and in interpreting the emotion conveyed by emoticons.

Keywords: Affect Analysis, Emoticon, Health and Fitness.

1 Introduction

Communication methods have greatly changed since the emergence of Web 2.0 technologies. The proliferation of text-based network applications, including e-mail, BBS (Bulletin Board Services), and instant messaging services have propelled the dissemination of ideas and knowledge. Although multimedia content including images, voice, and videos have also become prevalent in computer-mediated communication, text-based messages have not lost their popularity due to their convenience and compatibility between platforms. However, due to the lack of visual and vocal communication, text-based online communication suffers from the loss of non-verbal symbolic information, in comparison to face-to-face communication. As a compensation, symbols that mimic people's faces in order to express more nuanced opinions and emotions are often used along with text to aid in text-based communication. These symbols are called emoticons.

An emoticon is a metacommunicative pictorial representation of facial expression, which serves to convey information about the sender's emotional state. Emoticons

X. Zheng et al. (Eds.): ICSH 2014, LNCS 8549, pp. 1–12, 2014.
© Springer International Publishing Switzerland 2014

have been widely used by social media users and contribute to the facilitation of text-based communication technologies [3],[19]. Recently, we have observed an increasing use of emoticons in Chinese web forums and other social networking sites that feature health and fitness topics. The analysis of emoticons in these platforms can provide insights into how people use emoticons to express health-related concerns, and be considered a supplement to text-based affect analysis, since these symbols can reveal people's feelings and moods hidden beneath the text. For example, "Danced so far without being short of breath. Hooray sports and exercise! ~\(≧ ▽ ≦)/~" shows an exciting and happy mood, and "Finished the full course the first time. What should I do if have no strength to run tomorrow QAQ" shows an upset mood. As a result, a growing number of studies have started to examine the use of emoticons in social media. For instance, Ptaszynski et al. [16] used a kinesics-based approach for extraction and classification of emoticons, Tanaka et al. [20] used kernel methods and Yamada et al. [24] used n-grams statistics. However, very few works have investigated emoticons in a Chinese context or in health and fitness topics. Our work takes the first step in this area.

This paper presents a system which analyzes emoticons used in online discussions of Chinese health and fitness topics. The system extracts emoticons from posts and comments, and classifies them into one of the 7 pre-defined types automatically [2]. The system extracts semantic components (representations of eyes, mouth and other parts of human body) from emoticons and evaluates these areas integrally. The system utilizes a large lexicon of emotion symbols constructed based on existing online emoticon dictionaries, and adapts it to the Chinese context. The performance of the system is evaluated with empirical tests on a corpus of more than one million sentences of Chinese health and fitness topics.

The remainder of the paper is organized as follows. Section 2 provides a review of relevant literature and identifies potential research gaps. Section 3 presents our proposed Emoticon Analysis System framework. Section 4 describes our dataset and experiment settings, and discusses the results. Finally, section 5 concludes the study and identifies future directions.

2   Related Work

To form the basis of our research, we provide a review of recent emoticon studies. In general, four streams of emoticon research have been the most prevalent, which are discussed and summarized below.

2.1   Emoticon and User Behavior

The first stream of emoticon research focuses on the motivation of using emoticons, the outcomes of using emoticons, and how emoticons affect individuals' behaviors. For example, Rezabeck et al. [18] investigated the impact of emoticons in computer-mediated communication and concluded that emoticons helped clarify and enhance the meaning of text messages. Derks et al. [4] showed that people tend to use emoticons in a positive context and with their friends. Cao et al. [1] investigated emoticons in an online BBS, concluding that emoticons that could be easily inputted and intuitively understood are more frequently used by users. Wolf [23] pointed out the significant differences in the use of emoticons by men and women. Walther [22] concluded that emoticons' contributions were outweighed by verbal content, but a negativity effect appeared to shift message interpretation in the direction of the negative element. The above research has contributed valuable behavioral investigations into the pragmatics of emoticons used as a supplement of verbal language. However, these studies mostly focused on a small selected set of emoticons and their valence analysis, thus not concerning the variety of emoticons and the various emotions they conveyed.

2.2 Emoticon and Sentiment Analysis

The second stream of emoticon research focuses on using the valence of emoticons to improve classification performance in sentiment analysis. For example, Yang et al. [25] used emoticons to tag sentences appearing in articles, avoiding manual annotation. Poongodi et al. [15] and Jia et al. [7] proposed sentiment analysis models involving emoticons as features. Read [17] used emoticons to reduce topic dependency when using SVM classifiers for sentiment analysis. These studies confirmed the positive influence to involve emoticons in sentiment analysis. However, the coverage of emoticons was greatly limited, and the structure of emoticons was not thoroughly analyzed.

2.3 Emoticon Generation and Recommendation

This stream of studies focuses on emoticon generation and recommendation in human-computer interaction systems and input methods. Nakamura et al. [14] used a neural network-based algorithm to learn the relationship between sentences and emoticon areas (mouths, eyes) appearing in the sentences, and used them later to generate emoticons in a natural language dialogue system. Although the system occasionally generated strange emoticons, the idea of exploiting semantic areas of emoticons as base elements was enlightening.

Urabe et al. [21] focused on emoticon recommendation for Japanese computer-mediated communication. They first developed a text emotion analysis system to analyze the intended emotion from the emotional expressions used in the sentence, and then assisted the user in finding a suitable emoticon in an original emoticon database. They reported that the proposed system outperformed the existing system used in iPhones. Although we do not deal with emoticon recommendation, we found it useful to consider the emotional state of neighboring text when implementing emoticon classification.

2.4 Emoticon Extraction and Classification

This stream of studies aims to identify emoticons from text and classify emoticons into detailed affect categories (e.g., happiness, sadness, surprise, etc.). For example,

Tanaka et al. [20] used kernel methods for extraction and classification. They implemented the Dynamic Time Alignment Kernel (DTAK) and String Subsequence Kernel (SSK) in their SVM classifier. Yamada et al. [24] used statistics of n-grams on emoticon classification. They treated characters in emoticons as words in sentences, and concluded that the unigram method outperformed the bigram and trigram methods. Ptaszynski et al. [16] used a kinesics-based model on emoticon extraction and classification. They collected a large emoticon database from the Internet, divided the emoticons into semantic parts, and then classified them into emotion types. Their method adapted to users' creativity, using characters to construct new emoticons. However, the research above was conducted in a Japanese context. We need a system adaptable to Chinese, and confirm its validity for health and fitness topics.

2.5   Research Gaps and Questions

Based on the literature, several research gaps can be identified. Most prior studies focused on the emotion valence (i.e., positive or negative) carried by emoticons [7] [15] [17] [25], while emoticons contain richer semantics that express the affects of users, such as happiness, sorrow, and anger. For the studies focusing on emoticon affect extraction and refined classification [16] [20] [24], most were conducted in a Japanese context, which may not be directly applicable to a Chinese context or health and fitness topics.

In this study, we developed an emoticon analysis system to extract and classify text-based emoticons from Chinese texts related to health and fitness topics. We believe that these topics are important to society, and at the same time are important for young Chinese who actively use emoticons in social media. Specifically, we asked the following research questions:

• How can we effectively extract emoticons from Chinese texts?
• How accurate can we classify emoticons into different emotion types?

3   Research Design

Figure 1 illustrates the proposed dictionary-based emoticon extraction and classification system. The major components including Kinesics representation, affect mapping, emoticon extraction, and emoticon classification will be discussed in detail in the following subsections.

3.1   Kinesics Representation

The first step in our system was to develop a lexicon of emoticon symbols that could be used to suggest the meanings of new emoticons in Chinese texts. However, since we were not aware of any online resources for large-scale Chinese emoticon dictionary, we utilized several online Japanese emoticon dictionaries to construct the lexicon. The Japanese emoticon dictionaries included Face-mark Party [6], Kaomoji- café [8],

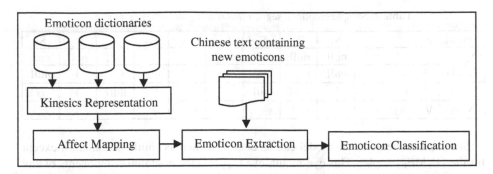

Fig. 1. Framework for extracting and classifying emoticons in Chinese text

Kaomoji Paradise [9], Kaomoji Station [10], Kaomojisyo [11], Kaomoji-toshokan [12], and Kaomojiya [13], which have been used by prior emoticon research [16]. Emoticons in these websites are already categorized with tags, such as "smile" or "cry." We only collected emoticons that were labeled by tags suggesting emotional meanings. Only categories with names suggesting emotional content were selected and emoticons from those categories were collected. In total, 11,988 emoticons were collected from the list of websites.

We observed that a large proportion of the collected emoticons contained Japanese Kana (a part of Japanese language), which is rarely seen in Chinese online social media and thus not adaptable to our Chinese context. Therefore, before using kinesics to represent the collected emoticons, we truncated Kana from raw emoticons. Table 1 shows several examples of this truncation process.

Table 1. Emoticon truncation

Emoticons before Truncation	Emoticons after Truncation
ヾ(>▽<)o きゃはははっ！	ヾ(>▽<)o
ムカ・・・(-_-メ)	(-_-メ)
キャハハハ!! ヾ(@⌒▽⌒@)ノ彡☆バンバン!!	ヾ(@⌒▽⌒@)ノ彡☆

Typically, emoticons convey emotions by mimicking people's faces. As a result, it is common that in an emoticon, some parts (character n-grams) represent people's eyes, some parts represent mouths, and so on. To segment emoticons into different semantic parts that represent different functional components, we adopted the kinesics model in Ptaszynski et al. [17] and represented each emoticon as the following 9 components:

$$\{S_1\}\{B_1\}\{S_2\}\{E_L\}\{M\}\{E_R\}\{S_3\}\{B_2\}\{S_4\}$$

where $\{B_1\}$ and $\{B_2\}$ are the borders of the emoticon (mostly parentheses), $\{E_L\}$ and $\{E_R\}$ are left and right eyes, $\{M\}$ is the mouth, and $\{S_1\}\{S_2\}\{S_3\}\{S_4\}$ are the remaining components representing other parts that can vary depending on context (e.g. sweat, arms, tool, breath, etc.). Table 2 presents some examples how emoticons are segmented into these 9 components.

Table 2. Sample emoticon segmentation using the kinesics model

Emoticon	S_1	B_1	S_2	E_L	M	E_R	S_3	B_2	S_4
＾_＾	null	null	null	＾	_	＾	null	null	null
(-_-ﾉ)	null	(	null	-	_	-	ﾉ	)	null
ヾ(>▽<)o	ヾ	(	null	>	▽	<	null	)	o
ヾ(@⌒▽⌒@)ﾉ彡	ヾ	(	@	⌒	▽	⌒	@	)	ﾉ彡

Some components in the model can be empty (shown as "null" in Table 2), except for the {E_LME_R} triplet. This eye-mouth-eye triplet is the essential components of any emoticon, and thus they were extracted as an integral part from the collected emoticons. Table 3 shows the number of distinct character sequences extracted for each component. From this table, we can see that {E_L}, {E_R}, and {M} were frequently reused in different emoticons, whereas the remaining components {S_1}{S_2}{S_3}{S_4} were more unique, especially for {S_4}. This suggested that people tended to describe their emotions more specifically by adding different characters after the {E_LME_R} triplet.

Table 3. Number of distinct character sequences extracted for each emoticon component

	Triplet	E_L	M	E_R	S_1	S_2	S_3	S_4
# of distinct char. sequences	3,518	343	623	339	1,704	1,444	1,405	4,109

3.2   Affect Mapping

Although the collected emoticons were already labeled with website-specific raw tags indicating their emotional meanings, such as "laughing" and "crying". These tags were often redundant and/or ambiguous. To suggest precise semantic meanings for new emoticons, they needed to be organized into distinct categories. One of the major emotional categorization schemas in psychology was proposed by Ekman et al. [5], who suggested a 6-type classification of affect categories: *happiness, sadness, fear, disgust, anger, and surprise*. In the Chinese context, Chen [2] suggested adding a seventh category, "*love*," into this categorization schema, extending it to a 7-type classification. Since the 7-type categorization contains two positive valence (i.e., happiness and love), it is considered to be more balanced in emoticon research. The original emotion tags in our collection also indicated that emoticons with a positive valence were more common than negative ones (as will be shown later). As a result, we adopted the 7-type categorization and mapped all the kinesics components into these 7 categories. The mapping process was started by manually categorizing all the raw tags into the 7 categories. All the emoticons belonging to a specific raw tag are then categorized accordingly. Table 4 shows the resulting categorization of all the collected dictionary emoticons.

We noticed that emoticons annotated as "happiness" accounted for approximately one third of the entire database, whereas the percentage was only 2.4% for "disgust"

Table 4. The number and percentage of emoticons in 7 affect categories

Affect Category	# of Emoticons	Percentage (%)
Happiness	3,879	32.4
Sadness	1,832	15.3
Fear	899	7.5
Anger	1,360	11.3
Disgust	286	2.4
Surprise	1,437	12.0
Love	2,295	19.1

category. This suggested that happiness was the most frequently expressed emotion by Internet users, whereas emoticons with "disgust" were not as popular as other emotion types. Overall, positive emotions (happiness and love) accounted for 51.5% and negative emotions (sadness, fear, anger, disgust and surprise) accounted for 48.5%, which indicated a relatively balanced distribution of emotion valence.

Furthermore, we separately mapped the $\{E_L M E_R\}$ triplets and $\{S_1\}\{S_2\}\{S_3\}\{S_4\}$ components into affect categories because the same triplet could be used to express different emotions. Table 5 shows several examples of how the same triplet could be assigned to different affect categories when other kinesics components were attached. We then counted how many times each triplet and component was assigned to each affect category, and used these numbers to model the probability of each triplet being used to express certain affects. In order to account for new Chinese emoticons containing triplets that did not exist in the constructed lexicon, we further separately modeled the possible affects of each individual part of a triplet $\{E_L\},\{M\}$, and $\{E_R\}$ using a similar process. These separately modeled triplets or single parts were used to infer the semantic meanings of new emoticons in the Chinese context.

Table 5. Examples of emoticon triplets associating with different affect categories

	Happiness	Sadness	Fear	Disgust	Anger	Surprise	Love
°Д°	(o°Д°o)	(ll°д°)	(*° д °)♂	ヾ(°д°;)	(#°Д°)	Σ(°Д°/)	l*°Д°Ħ
´艸`	(★´艸`)	-	-	-	-	(o·´艸`·)	-
·ω·	((p·ω·q))	(´·ω·`)	(/·ω··\)	-	-	Σ(·ω··;)	(*·ω·*)

3.3 Emoticon Extraction

To extract the emoticon strings from Chinese texts, we leveraged the construcuted emoticon symbol lexicon and compared the newly seen Chinese string and the triplets in our lexicon. If no match was found, the system further examined individual kinesics components to infer whether there were new triplets that did not exist in our lexicon, and tried to extract them. After the triplet was extracted, the system localized borders $\{B_1\}\{B_2\}$ in the input, which were usually parentheses, and then extracted additional components $\{S_1\}$ to $\{S_4\}$ from the input using regular expressions. The detailed procedure is described in the following pseudocode:

```
read(input)
output = emoticon_lexicon.find(input)
if output != null
    return output
end if
triplet = triplet_lexicon.find(input)
if triplet == null
    do
        (EL, M, ER) = individual_kinesics_component_lexicon.find(input)
        triplet = EL + M + ER
    until input.contains(triplet) or lexicon is traversalled
end if
if triplet == null
    return null
else
    (B1, B2) = localize_borders(input)
    regex = "(.*)" + B1 + "(.*)" + triplet + "(.*)" + B2 + "(.*)"
    (S1, S2, S3, S4) = regex.match(input)
end if
return output
```

3.4   Emoticon Classification

The emoticon classification was conducted based on the previous extraction procedure, where kinesics components $\{E_L M E_R\}$, $\{S_1\}$, $\{S_2\}$, $\{S_3\}$, $\{S_4\}$ were separately located in the extracted emoticon. We calculated the probability of each component being used to express certain affects from the lexicon, and inferred the type of the most probable affect which is expressed by the emoticon. The detailed procedure is described in the following pseudocode:

```
// triplet, S1, S2, S3, S4 are inherited from the previous extraction procedure
(happiness[0], sadness[0], fear[0], disgust[0], anger[0], surprise[0], love[0]) =
affect_category_frequency_for_triplets(triplet)
    for i = 1 to 4
        (happiness[i], sadness[i], fear[i], disgust[i], anger[i], surprise[i], love[i]) =
affect_category_frequency_for_si(s[i])
    end for
    largest_frequency = max(happiness[0~4], sadness[0~4], fear[0~4], disgust[0~4],
anger[0~4], surprise[0~4], love[0~4])
    for i = 0 to 4
```

```
     if largest_frequency == happiness[i]
          return "happiness"
     else if ... (omitted)
     else if largest_frequency == love[i]
          return "love"
     end if
end for
```

4   Test-Bed and Evaluations

4.1   Research Test-Bed

To test whether our proposed system was effective in detecting and classifying new emoticons in Chinese context, we collected comments and replies from two large, well-known Chinese video sites, (http://www.bilibili.tv) and (http://www.acfun.tv), which are popular among Chinese youngsters. Users upload their self-made videos onto these websites, sharing their creativity and mood with others. Specifically, we focused on videos belonging to food- and sports-related topics because we believe the majority of users interested in these topics are young, and we expected that a corpus with relatively rich emoticons could be obtained. In total, 1,003,244 comments were collected. They were posted for videos tagged by "food" or "sports" labels. Table 7 summarizes the statistics of our test-bed data.

Table 6. Test-bed statistics

# of comments	Acfun.tv	Bilibili.tv
Food related	463,434	215,144
Sports related	253,780	70,886

Within the test-bed, we manually annotated 2,000 comments, among which 985 contained emoticons. For these emoticons, we assigned one of the 7-type affect categories: happiness, sadness, fear, disgust, anger, surprise, or love. The rest of the comments were annotated as not containing emoticons. These annotated 2,000 comments were used as test dataset in emoticon extraction and classification tasks.

4.2   Evaluation of Emoticon Extraction Task

We evaluated the performance of our system on emoticon extraction by comparing the results of our system with the manual annotation on the test dataset. As a result, system precision was 99.4%, recall was 90.9%, and F-measure was 95.0%. Overall, the 95.0% F-measure indicated that our system was effective in extracting emoticons from Chinese text.

The very high precision rate indicated that emoticons often used very unique characters that were otherwise unused. Therefore, if any emoticon entry in our lexicon, including part of the emoticons (e.g. triplets), appeared in the given Chinese sentence, it was most likely used as an emoticon but not for any other purposes. The remaining

0.6% indicated that, however, there indeed existed some emoticons in the lexicon, but sometimes not used as emoticons in Chinese text. These were instead used as plain numbers or other characters. For example, "00" and "==" could both represent two eyes, or, respectively, could also appear in number "100" or be used as an equal sign.

The lower recall indicated that the system was weaker in recognizing visually similar but different characters. For example, "˘∀˘" and "˘○^" could not be properly recognized, although the lexicon contained numerous "∀˘" and "^O^" characters. Also, the system could not process characters that did not exist in the lexicon. These characters in most cases were unique to the Chinese encoding system, such as "‿ " and " ◡". To improve the system, these encoding problems must be addressed.

4.3   Evaluation on Emoticon Classification Task

In order to evaluate the effectiveness of the proposed system in classifying extracted emoticons, we compared our system with two benchmark classification systems used in prior research:

- Benchmark 1: classification based on the unigram model, implemented by Yamada et al. [24]. In this benchmark, the number of times each character was assigned to each affect category was counted without considering its position in the kinesics model, i.e. "o" in "^o^" and "o-o" are treated equally. This system considered the appearance frequency of each character in the lexicon and infers the affect category for the whole emoticon.
- Benchmark 2: classification based on only $\{E_L ME_R\}$ triplets. This benchmark system did not consider kinesics components $\{S_1\}\{S_2\}\{S_3\}\{S_4\}$ whenever a triplet was found, i.e. the triplet represents the whole emoticon, which was implemented by Ptaszynski et al. [16]. For example, after "˚Д˚" is found in "Σ(˚Д˚/)", "(#˚Д˚)" and "˵(˚Д˚;)", the system no longer considers "Σ", "/", "#", "˵" and ";", only analyzes the triplet as a result.

The emoticon classification tasks were performed on both the lexicon dataset and the manually annotated test dataset. The lexicon dataset included all 11,988 emoticons, which were mapped to the 7-type affect categories. The test-dataset included the 895 comments where emoticons were manually identified as present. Ten-fold cross-validation was conducted to compare the classification accuracy between different systems. Table 7 shows the classification results.

Table 7. Accuracy of emoticon classification tasks

Accuracy			
	Benchmark 1	Benchmark 2	Our system
Lexicon dataset	49.6%	69.5%	88.5%
Test dataset	40.3%	62.0%	73.1%
t-test value (H_0: Our system = benchmark)			
Lexicon dataset	57.98^{**}	12.00^{**}	-
Test dataset	6.18^{**}	2.42^{*}	-

*: p-value < 0.05; **: p-value < 0.01

The test results showed that our system significantly outperformed the two benchmarks, in both datasets. The relatively low accuracy for benchmark 1 suggested that a pure unigram algorithm was insufficient for describing the structure of emoticons. For example, the character "o" can be used as an eye, a mouth or a cheek, expressing different affects. Without specifying the character into detailed kinesics components, the affect it conveyed could not be properly analyzed. Benchmark 2 resulted in 62.0%~69.5 accuracy, still much lower than our system. This indicated that additional kinesics components $\{S_1\}$, $\{S_2\}$, $\{S_3\}$, and $\{S_4\}$ should be taken into consideration in addition to the eye-mouth-eye triplets. For example, " Σ (ﾟ Д ﾟ /)" was a surprised face, "(# ﾟ Д ﾟ)" an angry face and "ﾉ (ﾟ Д ﾟ ;)" a disgusted face. The triplets in these emoticons were identical ("ﾟ Д ﾟ"), thus the additional components " Σ ", "/", "#", "ﾉ", and ";" counted for their affect inclinations.

5   Conclusion and Future Directions

In this study, we developed an emoticon analysis system to extract and classify emoticons for Chinese text. Health and fitness-related online social media texts were used for empirical tests. We demonstrated that the kinesics model and the constructed emoticon lexicon helped improve the performance of emoticon extraction and classification tasks in Chinese context. We believe this work will expedite research on Chinese health and fitness topics, which is a less-explored and novel realm.

In this study, we examined only text-based emoticons, and did not include image-based emoticons which are also popular in online social media. Although adding the processing of images would demand the addition of computer image recognition technology, doing so may help resolve the system's weakness in recognizing visually similar characters. More advanced machine learning methods can also be implemented after achieving a deeper understanding of the structure of emoticons.

Acknowledgement. This study was supported by Chine Elite-1000 Program, Tsinghua University, USA NSF SES-1314631, and DUE-1303362. Also, the authors thank Cathy Larson for the proofreading and suggestions.

References

1. Cao, Z., Ye, J.: Attention Savings and Emoticons Usage in BBS. In: Proceedings of the Fourth International Conference on Computer Sciences and Convergence Information Technology (ICCIT 2009), pp. 416–419. IEEE (November 2009)
2. Chen, J.: The Construction and Application of Chinese Emotion Word Ontology. Master's Thesis, Dalian University of Technology, China (2009)
3. Chiu, K.C.: Explorations in the Effect of Emoticon on Negotiation Process from the Aspect of Communication. Master's Thesis, Department of Information Management, National Sun Yat-sen University, Taiwan (2007)
4. Derks, D., Bos, A.E., Grumbkow, J.V.: Emoticons and Social Interaction on the Internet: the Importance of Social Context. Computers in Human Behavior 23(1), 842–849 (2007)

5. Ekman, P.: Basic Emotions. In: Handbook of Cognition and Emotion, vol. 98, pp. 45–60 (1999)
6. Face-mark Party, http://www.facemark.jp/facemark.htm
7. Jia, S., Di, S., Fan, T.: Text Sentiment Analysis Model Based on Emoticons and Emotional Words. Journal of the Hebei Academy of Sciences 30(2), 11–15 (2013)
8. Kaomoji-café, http://kaomojicafe.jp/
9. Kaomoji Paradise, http://kaopara.net/
10. Kaomoji Station, http://kaosute.net/jisyo/kanjou.shtml
11. Kaomojisyo, http://matsucon.net/material/dic/
12. Kaomoji-toshokan, http://www.kaomoji.com/kao/text/
13. Kaomojiya, http://kaomojiya.com/
14. Nakamura, J., Ikeda, T., Inui, N., Kotani, Y.: Learning Face Marks for Natural Language Dialogue Systems. In: Proceedings of International Conference on Natural Language Processing and Knowledge Engineering, pp. 180–185. IEEE (October 2003)
15. Poongodi, S., Radha, N.: Classification of User Opinions from Tweets Using Machine Learning Techniques. International Journal of Advanced Research in Computer Science and Software Engineering 3(9) (2013)
16. Ptaszynski, M., Maciejewski, J., Dybala, P., Rzepka, R., Araki, K.: CAO: A Fully Automatic Emoticon Analysis System Based on Theory of Kinesics. IEEE Transactions on Affective Computing 1(1), 46–59 (2010)
17. Read, J.: Using Emoticons to Reduce Dependency in Machine Learning Techniques for Sentiment Classification. In: Proceedings of the ACL Student Research Workshop, pp. 43–48. Association for Computational Linguistics (June 2005)
18. Rezabek, L.L., Cochenour, J.J.: Visual Cues in Computer-Mediated Communication: Supplementing Text with Emoticons. Journal of Visual Literacy 18(2) (1998)
19. Suzuki, N., Tsuda, K.: Express Emoticons Choice Method for Smooth Communication of E-business. In: Gabrys, B., Howlett, R.J., Jain, L.C. (eds.) KES 2006, Part II. LNCS (LNAI), vol. 4252, pp. 296–302. Springer, Heidelberg (2006)
20. Tanaka, Y., Takamura, H., Okumura, M.: Extraction and Classification of Facemarks. In: Proceedings of the 10th International Conference on Intelligent User Interfaces, pp. 28–34. ACM (January 2005)
21. Urabe, Y., Rafal, R., Araki, K.: Emoticon Recommendation for Japanese Computer-Mediated Communication. In: Proceedings of the Seventh International Conference onSemantic Computing (ICSC), pp. 25–31. IEEE (September 2013)
22. Walther, J.B., D'Addario, K.P.: The Impacts of Emoticons on Message Interpretation in Computer-mediated Communication. Social Science Computer Review 19(3), 324–347 (2001)
23. Wolf, A.: Emotional Expression Online: Gender Differences in Emoticon Use. CyberPsychology & Behavior 3(5), 827–833 (2000)
24. Yamada, T., Tsuchiya, S., Kuroiwa, S., Ren, F.: Classification of Facemarks Using N-gram. In: Proceedings of International Conference on Natural Language Processing and Knowledge Engineering, pp. 322–327. IEEE (August 2007)
25. Yang, C., Lin, K.H., Chen, H.H.: Emotion Classification Using Web Blog Corpora. In: Proceedings of IEEE/WIC/ACM International Conference on Web Intelligence, pp. 275–278. IEEE (November 2007)

Diabetes-Related Topic Detection in Chinese Health Websites Using Deep Learning

Xinhuan Chen[1], Yong Zhang[1], Chunxiao Xing[1], Xiao Liu[2], and Hsinchun Chen[2]

[1] Research Institute of Information Technology,
Tsinghua National Laboratory for Information Science and Technology,
Department of Computer Science and Technology,
Tsinghua University, Beijing, China
xh-chen13@mails.tsinghua.edu.cn
{zhangyong05,xingcx}@tsinghua.edu.cn
[2] MIS Department, University of Arizona, United States
xiaoliu@email.arizona.edu, hchen@eller.arizona.edu

Abstract. With 98.4 million people diagnosed with diabetes in China, most of the Chinese health websites provide diabetes related news and articles in diabetes subsection for patients. However, most of the articles are uncategorized and without a clear topic or theme, resulting in time consuming information seeking experience. To address this issue, we propose an advanced deep learning approach to detect topics for diabetes related articles from health websites. Our research framework for topic detection on diabetes related articles in Chinese is the first one to incorporate deep learning in topic detection in Chinese. It can identify topics of diabetes articles with high performance and potentially assist health information seeking. To evaluate our framework, experiment is conducted on a test bed of 12,000 articles. The results showed the framework achieved an accuracy of 70% in detecting topics and significantly outperformed the SVM based approach.

Keywords: classification, topic detection, diabetes, Chinese, deep learning.

1   Introduction

Searching the Internet for health information has become increasingly common. A study in 2012 indicated that 80% of patients were interested in health-related information on the Internet [1]. Patients and their caregivers seek health-related information from the Internet for a variety of reasons. With the number of patients with chronic disease steadily growing every year, there is a severe shortage in health resources including nurses and physicians. Health professionals in China are often too busy to fully explain details of treatments and disease management to patients. Meanwhile, Internet provides accessible and comprehensive health information for patients. Convenience and privacy are also important reasons for patients to use the Internet, as they are not embarrassed to ask health questions online about their conditions.

According to the survey from the Chinese Diabetes Society, 98.4 million people were diagnosed with diabetes in China in 2013, more than any other country in the

X. Zheng et al. (Eds.): ICSH 2014, LNCS 8549, pp. 13–24, 2014.

world [2]. To meet the demand of health information from patients, many health-related websites were built in Chinese, providing services including health related news, articles, and health discussion boards. Articles from health websites contain abundant health information about diseases of interest contributed by both health professions and knowledgeable health consumers.

Although there is enormous amount of information available online, most of the articles are uncategorized. It is time-consuming and overwhelming for users to browse through a large number of articles and search for information about specific topics. Automatic topic detection from these articles could be important for both health consumers (e.g., patients and caregivers) and health professionals (e.g., physicians and nurses). It can provide health professionals and researchers with patients' discussion focus on the Internet. Moreover, topic detection can help health consumers, especially newly diagnosed patients to obtain valuable educational materials for their health self-management more efficiently.

Topic detection for health information has great potential to improve the efficiency of information seeking behaviors. However, little research has been done on Chinese context in this area. To address this issue, we propose an advanced deep learning approach to detect topics for diabetes related articles from health websites. Deep learning is an innovative machine learning approach for data analysis [3]. Witnessing outstanding performance in images and sound processing, deep learning has been incorporated in text mining to improve the performance recently [4, 5]. Our research framework for topic detection on diabetes related articles in Chinese is the first one to incorporate deep learning in topic detection in Chinese. It can identify topics with high performance and potentially assist health information seeking.

The rest of this paper is organized as follows. Section 2 provides a review of relevant literature. We describe our topic detection framework using deep learning in Section 3. Section 4 reports on our experiments and discusses the results. Finally, we conclude this paper in Section 5.

2   Related Work

To build the foundation of our study, we investigated current researches that conducted content analysis with online health information. Lu et al. [6] studied the content of three discussion boards on diabetes and cancer from an online health community. They found that health-related topics were discussed frequently. Other works focused on diabetes-related social networks. Weitzman et al. [7] analyzed ten diabetes-related websites and found that the quality of information was variable. Shrank et al. [8] manually reviewed content from 15 diabetes-related online social networks. Greene et al. [9] qualitatively analyzed the communications of Facebook communities dedicated to diabetes. They found one quarter of the posts were explicit advertisements, some of which advertised non-FDA (Food and Drug Administration) approved products, two-thirds were descriptions of personal experiences in diabetes management, and a quarter contained sensitive information unlikely to be revealed in doctor-patient interactions.

Topic discussions on health websites ranged from detailed symptoms to irrelevant spam. Several research methods have been adopted for topic detection in health websites. In earlier studies, topics of information offered by Internet medical support groups were determined based on the number of people who used the list and how frequently they posted [10]. Later, some researchers adopted questionnaires to statistically analyze interesting topics [11]. Li et al. [12] employed traditional statistical approaches to explore health-related topics. Lin et al. [13] applied an automatic document clustering method to categorize the retrieved literature into different topical groups and ranked the important literature in each group. In order to help diabetes patients find appropriate patient educational materials, Kandula et al. [14] proposed an approach to match education materials with patient clinical notes using topic modeling such that relevant education documents could be recommended to the patients. Brody et al. [15] used text classification based on the Latent Dirichlet Allocation (LDA) topic model to detect the salient topics of online health professionals' reviews.

Deep learning approaches are increasingly popular. Deep belief network (DBN) is a type of deep neural network, often adopted in image and text analysis. Tamilselvan et al. [16] presented a multi-sensor health diagnosis method using deep belief network (DBN). Wang et al. [17] used deep learning to analyze Chinese corpora and obtained satisfying results for automatic question-answering technique. Deep belief network have shown great potential to enhance the classification capability for complex medical Web articles. The following section describes in detail diabetes-related topic detection using DBN-based classification.

3   Research Design

3.1   Problem Definition

To better understand the topic detection, we provide a formal definition of our research problem as follow.

Definition 1. *Given the article collection* C *and category collection* T, *the labeled categories of each article* $d \in C$ *can be defined as*

$$L_d = [\, t_1, t_2, \ldots, t_i, \ldots, t_n], n \geq 1, t_i \in T$$

where t_1 is the primary category of each article.

Definition 2. *Given the article collection* C *and primary categories* P *of all the articles,* P $\sqsubseteq$ T; *topic* O *of each article* $d \in C$:

$$O_d \in P$$

O_d is the output of our topic detection framework for each diabetes-related article.

3.2   Topic Detection Framework

We propose a framework to automatically determine diabetes-related topics of articles from Chinese health websites. Our framework includes four components: data collection, data preprocessing, training the DBN model, and topic classification, as shown in Figure 1.

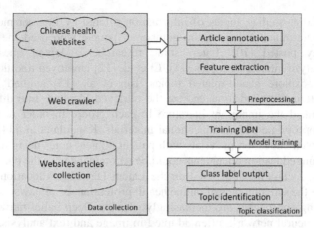

Fig. 1. Topic detection framework

Data Collection

We developed an automated crawler to download Web pages from Chinese health websites. Keywords were used to help identify diabetes-related pages. Text parsers were used to extract specific fields including ID, URL, title, source, post time, message body content, and tags from the web pages and store in our data repository. Message body contents are the major focus in this study. Further, extracted tags can be used as a reference to diabetes categorization. We collected 11,216 articles to form our test bed.

Data Preprocessing

Data preprocessing is a critical component for further analysis. The process consists of five steps: dictionary acquisition, word segmentation, categorization, article annotation, and feature extraction.

To build a diabetes domain specific lexicon for this study, we combined entries from Diabetes Dictionary App[1], a commercial mobile application for diabetes patients, and the keyword tags from diabetes-related web pages to form a relatively comprehensive Chinese diabetes lexicon. We used ICTCLAS[2], a Chinese word segmentation tool developed by the Chinese Academy of Science, to remove stop words and perform word segmentation for the body contents of pages.

We summarized the diabetes categories in Figure 2. We created six primary categories that describe different aspects of diabetes. This diagram contains three levels of sub-categories. We collected 50 categories in total. Due to space limitations, some sub-categories are not shown in Figure 2. Some sub-categories may have multiple parent categories. "Fruit," for instance, shown under the main category of "Diabetes care" (subcategory, "Diabetes diet"), also fits under the main category of "Diabetes prevention."

---

[1] http://as.baidu.com/a/item?docid=1018036888&f=web_am_rel
[2] http://ictclas.org/

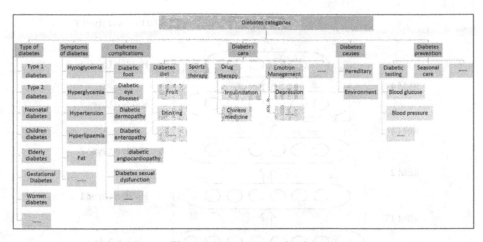

Fig. 2. Diabetes categorization

Once we completed the diabetes categorization, we manually annotated and labeled each article. Each article was assigned one main label but may have been assigned one or more secondary labels.

We then extracted the feature vectors as the input nodes of the DBN. Bag-of-words (BOW) is often adopted as features for deep learning. However, it can result in a large but sparse feature set. High dimensional feature vectors with only several non-zero values affect the performance of DBN model [20]. To reduce the dimensionality of the feature vectors, we developed a feature set containing 1065 diabetes related words from the diabetes lexicon. Finally, each article was presented as a vector with 1065 dimensions. All features were binary, denoting whether the corresponding word appeared in the article or not.

Model Training
The DBN model is described in Section 3.3. The feature vectors served as the input nodes in the visible layer of DBN. The network output 50 probability values of nodes representing the article main categories.

Topic Classification
The labels of the maximum probability value can be used for articles classification. Once the label was obtained, the higher level categories were checked through a category tree structure as shown in Figure 2. The diabetes-related topic belonging to the six first level categories was identified.

3.3   Deep Belief Network

DBN uses a multilayered architecture that consists of one visible layer and multiple hidden layers as shown in Figure 3. In order to facilitate the learning process, the visible layer of a DBN accepts the input data and transfers the data to the hidden layers [18]. DBN uses RBMs (Restricted Boltzmann Machine) as the building blocks for each layer [19].

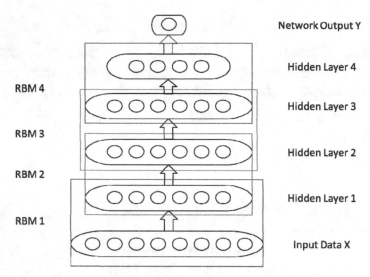

Fig. 3. Deep belief network architecture

Each RBM consists of two layers, the visible layer and the hidden layer. The connections between the nodes with each RBM layer (from visible layer to hidden layer) are finished through an activation function based on the RBM learning rule. The DBN consists of four stacked RBMs: the input data layer and hidden layer 1 form the first RBM, continuous hidden layers form the next RBM, and the final output layer is reserved for the next step of the DBN training.

DBN models the joint distribution between visible vector x and the k-th hidden layer h^k as follows [5]:

$$p(x, h^1, \dots, h^k) = \left(\prod_{k=0}^{K-2} p(h^k | h^{k+1}) \right) \cdot p(h^{K-1}, h^K) \tag{1}$$

where x is the input data vector, $p(h^k | h^{k+1})$ is a conditional distribution for visible nodes conditioned on the hidden nodes of the RBM at layer k, and $p(h^{K-1}, h^K)$ is the visible-hidden joint distribution in the top-level RBM. The process of layer-wise unsupervised training can be described as follows:

1. Train the first layer as an RBM that models the raw input x as its visible layer.
2. Use the first layer to obtain a representation of the input that will be used as data for the second layer. This representation can be chosen as the mean activation of $p(h^1 = 1|x)$.
3. Train the second layer as an RBM, taking the transformed data (mean activation) as training examples.
4. Iterate 2 and 3 for the desired number of layers, each time propagating upward samples.
5. Fine-tune all the parameters of the deep architecture with respect to a proxy for the DBN log-likelihood, or with respect to a supervised training method (becoming supervised predictions, e.g., a linear classifier).

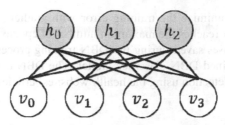

Fig. 4. RBM graphical depiction

Each RBM consists of two layers as shown in Figure 4. There are a number of nodes in each layer and there is no weight connection between nodes with the same layer [19]. Thus, the training parameters in a RBM contain the weights between layers and the node biases. The states of nodes in the RBM hidden layer are determined through transforming the states of nodes of the visible layer with an activation function. Each training epoch consists of two phases. The first phase transforms the input data from the visible layer to the hidden layer and the second phase operates as a reconstruction of the nodes of the previous visible layer. The process can be expressed as follows:

$$p(h^k = 1|v) = sigmoid(-b_k - \sum_j v_j w_{kj}) \qquad (2)$$

$$p(v^j = 1|h) = sigmoid(-b_j - \sum_k h_k w_{kj}) \qquad (3)$$

where sigmoid activation function is shown as:

$$sigmoid(\mathrm{x}) = 1/(1 + e^{-x}) \qquad (4)$$

where h^k and v^j are the states for the k-th node in hidden layer and the j-th node in the visible layer, respectively. The visible and hidden layers nodes are binary stochastic variables with values 0 or 1, representing off or on condition of the nodes in the learning process.

We then update parameters (weights w_{kj} and biases b_j) based on state vectors of nodes in both the hidden and visible layers. The update of weights w_{jk} can be formulated as

$$\Delta w_{jk} = \varepsilon(< v_j h_k >_{data} - < v_j h_k >_{recon}) \qquad (5)$$

where ε is the learning rate between 0 and 1, $< v_j h_k >_{data}$ is the pairwise product of the state vectors for first phase, whereas $< v_j h_k >_{recon}$ denotes the pairwise product for reconstruction of the visible layer. The same update rule is used for biases. The training parameters such as weights and biases of each RBM in a DBN architecture are continuously updated until a maximum number of training epochs is reached.

After all RBMs finish the training process, the DBN can fine-tune all the parameters of the deep architecture with respect to a supervised training method, which is accomplished by the back-propagation algorithm. The back-propagation learning process considers all layers simultaneously, and the training error is calculated using network outputs and the target data labels. All parameters of the

DBN are updated to minimize the training error with gradient descent. The process stops when the network reaches the maximum number of epochs.

The weights and biases saved during the DBN training process are used to test the performance of the trained DBN classifier model. The DBN can then be applied for diabetes-related topic detection using the health websites' articles.

4   Experiments

4.1   Test Bed

To evaluate the performance of the topic detection framework, we developed a research test bed with articles from diabetes sub-sections in two Chinese health websites[3]. A summary of the test bed is shown in Table 1.

Table 1. Dataset summary

Websites name	tnbz.com	zzcxhg.com
Number of articles	4,193	7,023
Sample articles	糖尿病患者大多听说,粥是喝不得的,会使血糖迅速上升。治疗糖尿病的医生们,也多把吃干不吃稀当成铁律告诫糖尿病患者。肥胖者也会听说:喝粥容易消化,容易饥饿,越喝越胖。这些说法是否完全正确呢?恐怕非常值得商榷。一篇广为流传的文章谈到:有研究发现,等量大米煮成的米饭或粥对糖尿病患者进食后血糖有不同的影响。⋯⋯ Most diabetes patients hear that they cannot eat porridge, which can make blood sugar rise rapidly. The doctors also tell patients not to eat porridge. Obese people also hear that porridge is easy to digest and get hungry. The more one drinks the more weight he or she gains. Is it quite right? A widely circulated article said that one study found that the same amount of rice and porridge have different effects on diabetes blood sugar after eating.	一个研究报告称,在预防糖尿病心血管并发症方面,绝对素食者饮食比美国糖尿病协会推荐的饮食更有益。大约2/3的糖尿病患者死于心脏病或者是中风,因此预防心血管的发病是重中之重。这个研究由美国医师委员会资助,该委员会倡议绝对素食者饮食。⋯⋯ According to a research report, vegan diet is more helpful than the American diabetes association recommends eating in the prevention of cardiovascular complications in diabetes. About two-thirds diabetes patients die of heart disease and stroke. Thus the prevention of cardiovascular disease is a top priority. The study was funded by the U.S. physicians' committee, the committee suggests vegan diet.

---

[3] http://www.tnbz.com/
   http://www.zzcxhg.com/

Table 1. (*continued*)

Number of distinct tags	888	49
Number of all tags	6,933	7,023
Examples of tags	高饱腹感;低血糖反应 high satiety, hypoglycemia	饮食控制 diet control
Time span		[2010-07-06,2013-9-18]
Total number of distinct tags		912
Total number of articles		11,216
Average number of annotated articles per category		224.32

We labeled all articles with the 50 categories shown in Figure 2. The distribution of articles over all the categories is shown in Figure 5. The distribution was very unbalanced: 9 classes contained fewer than 10 articles as shown in Figure 5. We investigated the classes and found that these class labels were about rare complications, such as diabetes breast cancer, hyperlipaemia, diabetic hepatopathy, diabetic neurogenic bladder disease, and diabetes bone disease. 6 classes contained more than 500 articles with categories such as diabetes care, symptoms of diabetes, diabetes diet and diabetes prevention.

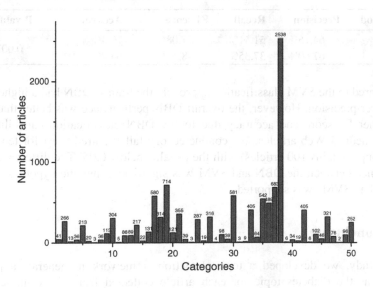

Fig. 5. The number of articles over all categories

4.2   Evaluation Metrics

We adopted standard machine learning evaluation metrics accuracy, precision, recall and F1 score[4] to evaluate the performance of the DBN classification. These metrics have been widely used in data mining studies [16].

4.3   Baseline

To demonstrate the performance of our DBN based topic detection framework, we adopted SVM classification model as the baseline for comparison. Support Vector Machine is one of the most popular and effective text classification techniques and has been adopted in medical research [18]. The SVM constructs hyper-planes with maximum margins to divide data points with different class labels. We adopted libSVM[5], an open source software package for the experiment.

4.4   Results and Analysis

The test bed has 11,165 diabetes related articles, each of which has been assigned a category after manual annotation. We divided the dataset into two sets; the training set contained 10,165 articles, and testing set contained 1,000 articles. Table 2 shows the performance of topic detection on diabetes related articles.

Table 2. Evaluation of Topic Detection

Method	Precision	Recall	F1 score	Accuracy	P-value
DBN	64.15%	51.41%	57.08%	70.4%	0.007998
SVM	67.60%	37.35%	48.11%	63.2%	

Compared to the SVM classification approach, the trained DBN had a higher recall but a lower precision. However, the overall DBN performance was better than SVM with higher F1 score and accuracy due to the DBN classification capability with complex medical Web articles. We conducted one tailed paired t-test for ten groups (each group contains 100 articles) with the p-value below 0.05. The difference of the performance between the DBN and SVM was significant, thus the hypothesis "DBN is better than SVM" was supported.

5   Conclusion

In this study, we developed a topic detection framework to generate a primary category as the diabetes topic for each article collected from the Chinese health websites. This framework included four components: data collection, data preprocessing, training DBN model, and topic classification. The DBN model

---

[4] http://en.wikipedia.org/wiki/F1_score
[5] http://www.csie.ntu.edu.tw/~cjlin/libsvm/

enhanced the classification capability for complex Chinese diabetes articles. The experimental results showed that the DBN outperformed state-of-the-art text classification techniques for diabetes-related articles. In the future, we will explore other chronic diseases in Chinese health websites.

Acknowledgements. The work described in this paper was supported by grants from the National Basic Research Program of China (973 Program) No. 2011CB302302, the 1000-Talent program, and the Tsinghua University Initiative Scientific Research Program.

References

1. Monnier, J., Laken, M., Carter, C.L.: Patient and Caregiver Interest in Internet-Based Cancer Services. Cancer Practice 10(6), 305–310 (2002)
2. Chinese Diabetes Society,
   http://cdschina.org/news_show.jsp?id=2121.html
3. Deep Learning Tutorials by LISA lab,
   http://www.deeplearning.net/tutorial/
4. Socher, R., Bengio, Y., Manning, C.D.: Deep learning for NLP (without magic).Tutorial Abstracts of ACL. p. 5. Association for Computational Linguistics (2012)
5. Gouws, S.: Deep unsupervised feature learning for natural language processing. In: Proceedings of the 2012 Conference of the North American Chapter of the Association for Computational Linguistics, pp. 48–53 (2012)
6. Lu, Y., Zhang, P., Liu, J., et al.: Health-related hot topic detection in online communities using text clustering. PloS One 8(2), e56221 (2013)
7. Weitzman, E.R., Cole, E., Kaci, L., et al.: Social but safe? Quality and safety of diabetes-related online social networks. JAMIA 18(3), 292–297 (2011)
8. Shrank, W.H., Choudhry, N.K., Swanton, K., et al.: Variations in structure and content of online social networks for patients with diabetes. Archives of Internal Medicine 171(17), 1589–1591 (2011)
9. Greene, J.A., Choudhry, N.K., Kilabuk, E., et al.: Online social networking by patients with diabetes: a qualitative evaluation of communication with Facebook. Journal of General Internal Medicine 26(3), 287–292 (2011)
10. Klemm, P., Nolan, M.T.: Internet cancer support groups: legal and ethical issues for nurse researchers. Oncology Nursing Forum 25(4), 673–676 (1998)
11. Basch, E.M., Thaler, H.T., Shi, W., et al.: Use of information resources by patients with cancer and their companions. Cancer 100(11), 2476–2483 (2004)
12. Li, N., Wu, D.D.: Using text mining and sentiment analysis for online forums hotspot detection and forecast. Decision Support Systems 48(2), 354–368 (2010)
13. Lin, Y., Li, W., Chen, K., et al.: A document clustering and ranking system for exploring MEDLINE citations. JAMIA 14(5), 651–661 (2007)
14. Kandula, S., Curtis, D., Hill, B., et al.: Use of topic modeling for recommending relevant education material to diabetic patients. In: AMIA, vol. 2011, p. 674 (2011)
15. Brody, S., Elhadad, N.: Detecting salient aspects in online reviews of health providers. In: AMIA, vol. 2010, p. 202 (2010)
16. Tamilselvan, P., Wang, P.: Failure diagnosis using deep belief learning based health state classification. Reliability Engineering & System Safety 115, 124–135 (2013)

17. Wang, B., Liu, B., Wang, X., et al.: Deep learning approaches to semantic relevance modeling for chinese question-answer pairs. TALIP 10(4), 21 (2011)
18. Hinton, G.E., Osindero, S., Teh, Y.W.: A fast learning algorithm for deep belief nets. Neural Computation 18(7), 1527–1554 (2006)
19. Hinton, G.: A practical guide to training restricted Boltzmann machines. Momentum 9(1), 926 (2010)
20. Salakhutdinov, R., Hinton, G.: Semantic hashing. International Journal of Approximate Reasoning 50(7), 969–978 (2009)

Identifying Adverse Drug Events from Health Social Media: A Case Study on Heart Disease Discussion Forums

Xiao Liu[1], Jing Liu[2], and Hsinchun Chen[1]

[1] Artificial Intelligence Lab, University of Arizona, United States
xiaoliu@email.arizona.edu, hchen@eller.arizona.edu
[2] School of Management, Northwestern Polytechnical University, China
liujing2968@gmail.com

Abstract. Health social media sites have emerged as major platforms for discussions of treatments and drug side effects, making them a promising source for listening to patients' voices in adverse drug event reporting. However, extracting patient adverse drug event reports from social media continues to be a challenge in health informatics research. To utilize the fertile health social media data for drug safety research, we develop advanced information extraction techniques for identifying adverse drug events in health social media. A case study is conducted on a heart disease discussion forum to evaluate the performance. Our approach achieves an f-measure of 82% in the recognition of medical events and treatments, an f-measure of 69% for identifying adverse drug events and an f-measure of 90% in patient report extraction. Analysis on the extracted adverse drug events suggests that health social media can provide supplemental information for adverse drug events and drug interactions. It provides a less biased insight into the distribution of adverse events among heart disease population compared to data from a drug regulatory agency.

Keywords: Health social media analytics, Adverse drug event extraction, Statistical learning, Medical entity extraction, Heart disease.

1 Introduction

According to the annual report from the US Centers for Disease Control and Prevention (CDC), in 2012 there were 25.6 million diagnosed heart disease patients in the United States. Much of the population is at risk of developing heart disease. There is an estimated 154.7 million overweight and obese US adults and 78 million adults have hypertension, all of which are important risk factors for heart disease. Reducing mortality and morbidity of heart disease is a major focus of current American healthcare.

Patients with heart disease are particularly vulnerable to adverse drug events (ADE) due to their advanced age, polypharmacy, and the influence of heart disease on drug metabolism. Approximately 1% of the adverse drug events experienced by heart

X. Zheng et al. (Eds.): ICSH 2014, LNCS 8549, pp. 25–36, 2014.

disease patients are considered severe, requiring immediate clinical intervention [1]. The ADE potential for a particular heart disease drug varies with the individual, the disease being treated, and the extent of exposure to other drugs. Thus, listening to patients' speak about their heart disease medication experience and identifying adverse drug events is critical to improve patient safety and reduce mortality and morbidity.

Although adverse drug events should be reported through available channels such as the FDA's Adverse Event Reporting System, many patients do not do so, perhaps because of ignorance of these channels, perceptions of negative provider attitude, or extreme illness [2]. Instead, they often use online patient discussion forums and social networks to share an adverse drug event experience with other patients. As a result, online discussion forums and social websites can provide a fertile data source for researchers and health professionals to identify and evaluate adverse drug events [3].

Mining patient social media for adverse drug events can help healthcare practitioners to understand patients' concerns and problems; thus it has the potential to improve patient safety [4]. To date, there is little research that applies information extraction techniques to identify and analyze heart disease-related adverse drug events in patient social media. This is a challenging task as there are multiple types of drug-related discussions confounded with patient adverse drug event reports. Table 1 shows sample posts from one heart disease forum.

Table 1. Sample posts from a heart disease forum

Post ID	Sentence	Relation Type
217542	No anti angina [Drug] treatment because allergy [Event] to nitrates?	ADE
20473	I was taking Hyzaar [Drug] and Norvasc [Drug] for hypertension [Event].	Drug Indication
84495	It is true the beta blocker [Drug] maintains a lower heart rate, but it also stabilizes the heart rate to prevent arrhythmia [Event].	Prevention
8309	I have never [Negation] had dizziness [Event] from Warfarin[Drug].	Negated ADE
236521	If they essentially appear with low heart rate [Event], beta blockers [Drug] usually don't work.	Others

The relation types of co-occurred drug and medical events in heart disease treatments include adverse drug event, negated adverse drug event, drug indication, prevention and other relations. Adverse drug event describes a drug and a side effect caused by the drug. Negated adverse drug event denies the causal relationship between the drug and event. Drug indication presents a drug and a medical condition for which the drug is prescribed. Prevention represents a relation between a drug and a medical event which the drug is used to prevent. In other cases, there might be no causal relationship between the use of a drug and a medical event.

Given the great potential of health social media content and the challenge of identifying adverse drug events from this new emerging data source, we are motivated to develop advanced information extraction techniques for identifying and analyzing adverse drug event reports in heart disease discussion forums.

2   Related Work

A large number of health social media platforms are available on the Internet and have been explored in prior research in this area. These platforms can be categorized as general health discussion forums such as DailyStrength and MedHelp [4-7], disease-focused discussion forums for diabetes and breast cancer [2,3,8] and microblogs (Twitter) [9].

The most commonly adopted information extraction techniques in health social media research include text classification, medical entity recognition and adverse drug event extraction. Text classification has been applied in health social forums to filter noise [9], to classify positive or negative drug effects [4] and to extract ADE reports based on patient experience [8]. Support Vector Machines (SVM), one of the most popular ways to perform text classification, is widely adopted in past studies [4,8,9].

Medical entity extraction is a common way to extract user comments related to drugs and adverse events. Most studies adopt lexicon-based entity extraction because of the wide availability of medical lexicons in the healthcare domain. These lexicons include the Unified Medical Language System(UMLS), a medical knowledge base from the National Library of Medicine [2,4,5,8] , Drug Safety databases such as FAERS, the FDA's Adverse Event Reporting System [8,9], MedEffect, an adverse drug event report database from Canada [4,5] and SIDER, a side effect resource based on information extracted from package inserts [4,5]. Consumer Health Vocabulary (CHV), a lexicon linking UMLS standard medical terms to health consumer vocabulary, has also been applied in prior studies to better understand and match user expressions in social media [2,7,8]. Nikfarjam et al. [6] adopted a machine-learning approach with association rule mining to find patterns for adverse reactions mentioned in annotated data.

Adverse drug event extraction is an application of relation extraction, which scans text for relations between drugs and medical events and extracts adverse drug event relations. ADE extraction techniques can be categorized into three different approaches: co-occurrence analysis, rule-based and statistical learning. In prior studies, the co-occurrence-based approach has been predominantly used to extract drug and adverse event relations from user comments because of its simplicity and flexibility [2,3,4,6,7,8]. This approach assumes that if two entities co-occur within a certain distance, there is an underlying relationship between them [2]. Lately, more sophisticated relation extraction techniques, such as rule-based and statistical learning approaches, have been adopted in adverse drug event extraction [8]. Liu et al. [8] developed a hybrid adverse drug event extraction technique consisting of statistical learning-based relation extraction to identify related drug and event pairs and rule-based relation classification to extract adverse drug event pairs from all related drug and event pairs.

Several studies have evaluated their performance on extracting medical entities in social media [5,6,8]. Leaman et al. [5] obtained the best performance with an f-measure of 74% in extracting adverse event entities using a lexicon-based approach. Liu et al. [8] obtained an f-measure of 92% in extracting drug named entities and an f-measure of 83% in extracting medical event entities. However some of these medical events are drug indications, not necessarily adverse events. For adverse drug event extraction, Liu et al. [8] examined the hybrid approach with both statistical learning and rule-based filtering. Their approach achieved 82% in precision, 56% in recall and 67% in f-measure, which significantly outperformed the co-occurrence-based approach. For text classification, Bian et al. [9] achieved 74% accuracy in identifying ADE related tweets, and Liu et al. [8] achieved an f-measure of 84% in identifying patient reports of ADEs.

An information extraction framework which consists of lexicon-based medical entity extraction, a hybrid approach with statistical learning and rule-based filtering for ADE extraction and text classification to extract reports based on patients' accounts has been proved with satisfying performance in a diabetes forum dataset [8]. However, the effectiveness of this approach on datasets that have more complex relation types hasn't been tested. Although several disease-focused discussion forums have been adopted as test beds to conduct in-depth analysis on patient-reported adverse drug events for specific diseases including breast cancer and diabetes, there is no prior study that emphasizes heart disease adverse drug events, which is a major chronic disease in the United States.

Based on the review of prior studies, we proposed the following research question: How can we develop a high performance information extraction framework for mining patient-reported adverse drug events from heart disease forums?

3   Research Design

We discuss our proposed adverse drug event extraction framework in this section. The framework includes patient forum data collection, preprocessing, medical entity extraction, adverse drug event extraction, and report source classification.

3.1   Patient Forum Data Collection

Heart disease-related social media discussion was collected from MedHelp, a general health discussion forum, using a web crawler. We developed a java-based text parser to extract specific fields from the downloaded HTML pages. These fields include post ID (the unique identifier of a post), user profile, user name, topic ID, topic title, board ID, URL, post date and content.

3.2   Preprocessing

For data preprocessing, we developed regular expression-based text cleaning procedures to remove URL, duplicated punctuation, telephone number, SSN and other personal identifiable information. We conducted sentence boundary detection to segment posts into sentences so the data would be suitable for subsequent analysis.

3.3   Lexicon-Based Medical Entity Extraction

Due to the wide availability of medical lexicons and their satisfying performance in prior studies, we adopted a lexicon-based approach for medical entity extraction. Specifically, we utilized MetaMap [10] to extract mentions of drugs and medical events. The professional terms that never appear in FAERS reports were filtered out. Considering the diverse colloquial expressions in forum discussions, we expanded our medical lexicon with colloquial terms from the Consumer Health Vocabulary corresponding to standard medical terms extracted by MetaMap.   Based on the results of medical entity extraction, we selected sentences with both drug mentions and medical events for further analysis.

3.4   Adverse Drug Event Extraction

Adverse drug event extraction can be formulated as a relation extraction task. There are two subtasks: relation detection and relation classification.

Relation detection aims to detect whether a drug and a medical event in the same sentence are related. We utilized the Stanford Parser[1] to generate the shortest dependency path between the drug and event and added syntactic classes (Part-of-speech tags and generalized part-of-speech tags) and semantic classes (Treatment and Event) to expand the feature set. The shortest dependency path kernel was applied to conduct relation detection [11]. Transductive SVM-light [12], an open source software package for SVM, was adopted for semi-supervised learning from both labeled and unlabeled data.

We developed a rule-based relation classification algorithm to extract adverse drug events from all related drug and event pairs. The types of relations considered in our research include: adverse drug event, drug indication, prevention and negated adverse drug event. We utilized NegEx [13] and FAERS to filter out negated adverse drug event and drug indication respectively. We developed relation patterns based on a set of signaling words including 'prevent', 'avoid', 'circumvent the possibility', 'reduce the risk', 'reduce the chance of ', 'decrease the risk' and 'decrease the chance' to filter out relations related to prevention.

3.5   Report Source Classification

We developed a feature-based classifier to distinguish patient reports from hearsay and generated 7,416 features by combining bag-of-words (BOW) and Part-of-speech (POS) tags. We removed stop words, converted all characters to lower case and replaced all numbers with a "D" to reduce the feature sparsity. Transductive SVM-light with linear kernel was adopted for semi-supervised learning-based report source classification.

---

[1] Stanford Parser: http://nlp.stanford.edu/software/
stanford-dependencies.shtml/

3.6   Research Hypotheses

Based on the related literature review and our research question, the following hypotheses are proposed.

H1. Statistical learning-based adverse drug event extraction in patient forums can outperform co-occurrence analysis-based approaches.

H1a. Rule-based adverse drug event extraction will outperform co-occurrence-based approaches.

H1b. Conducting relation detection before relation classification will outperform direct relation classification models.

H2. Report source classification can improve the results of patient adverse drug event report extraction as compared to not accounting for report source issues.

4   Experiments

4.1   Test Bed

To verify the effectiveness of our framework, we investigated the forum discussions in a well-known online health community, MedHelp. We selected three of the most popular heart disease discussion boards. A summary of the test bed and detailed statistics are illustrated in Table 2.

Table 2. Test bed forum boards

Board	# of Posts	# of Topics	Time Span	# of Sentences
Heart Disease Community	166,213	48,451	1995/1/1-2014/1/8	1,423,379
Heart Rhythm Community	84,896	17,460	2007/6/1-2014/1/10	691,545
Coronary Heart Disease (CAD) Community	363	101	2007/3/3-2014/1/10	3,177

4.2   Evaluation Metrics

We used standard machine-learning evaluation metrics, accuracy, precision, recall and f-measure, to evaluate the performance of medical entity extraction, adverse drug event extraction and report source classification. These metrics have been widely used in information extraction studies [4,5,6,8].

4.3   Evaluation

To build a gold standard for evaluation, we manually annotated 250 sentences with both drug and event entities, including 462 drug and event pairs and 350 randomly selected sentences with one drug or event term or without any medical entity. The detailed distribution is shown in Table 3.

Table 3. Distribution of entities, relations and report source in annotated data

Entity Type	# of Mentions	Relation Type	# of Occurrences
Drug	321	Has Relation	324
Event	343	ADE	136
Report Source	*# of Sentences*	Drug Indication	156
Patient Experience	160	Negated ADE	5
Hearsay	90	Prevention	22
		Others	5
		No Relation	138

The medical entity extraction performance was evaluated by comparing the lexicon-based extraction results to manual annotation. The results of the evaluation are shown in Table 4.

Table 4. Medical entity extraction evaluation

Entity	Precision	Recall	F-measure
Drug	94.29%	81.32%	87.33%
Event	79.30%	73.25%	76.16%

Drug entity extraction achieved an f-measure of 87.33%. For medical event extraction, our system achieves an f-measure of 76.16%. This performance is slightly lower than that of the prior study on a diabetes discussion forum [8]. MedHelp is a general health discussion forum, which consists of more than one hundred discussion boards for different diseases, has more diverse participants and more linguistic diversity in discussion than the diabetes forum. The low recalls for both drug and adverse event entity extraction are mainly attributed to spelling errors in the posts. This kind of error can be lessened by using more robust string matching techniques. Colloquial expressions in online communities affect the low recall for medical event extraction. This kind of error can be relieved by applying semantic analysis to the sentences and building more context-dependent lexicons. Table 5 lists examples of errors in medical entity extraction.

Table 5. Examples of errors in medical entity extraction

Error Type	Post	Sentence	Error
Drug spelling error	2085	They tell me no more room for stents, the meds are **atenoteol** 20mg, amlodipine 5mg, losartan 5mg, plavix 75 mg, Crestor 40 mg, Asprine 81mg?	"atenoteol" -> "atenolol"
Event spelling error	15253	I am already experiencing when I have these **palpatations** for any length of time	"palpatations" -> "palpitations"
Colloquial expression	41235	He is a diabetic (type 2) non-ischemic DCM/CHF patient hampered by episodes (minutes to hours) of dullness, low energy, weakness, and **feeling need of 'deep breaths'**.	"feeling need of 'deep breaths'"-> "short of breath"
	41126	I have been on Pristiq for 3 yrs, all of a sudden the nausea, dizziness, dry mouth, lots of diarrhea, fatigue, **lost 49 lbs**, insomnia, irritability, vertigo, terrible dreams.	"lost 49 lbs" -> "weight loss"

We annotated 462 drug-event pairs from the 18,865 pairs. The distributions of all relation types are illustrated in Table 3. To minimize the influence of variability in the training set, we conducted 5-fold cross validation for adverse drug event extraction. We evaluated our kernel-based relation detection with rule-based relation classification (RD+RC) against the results from co-occurrence analysis (CO) and rule-based relation classification (RC). As illustrated in Table 6, kernel-based relation detection combined with rule-based relation classification (RD+RC) performs best with 65.36% precision and 73.53% recall. Compared to co-occurrence, direct rule-based relation classification (RC) yields higher precision but lower recall. Overall, rule-based performance is better than the co-occurrence-based approach.

Table 6. Results of Adverse Drug Event Extraction

Method	Accuracy	Precision	Recall	F-measure
CO	29.44%	29.44%	100%	45.49%
RC	63.20%	42.74%	73.53%	54.06%
RD+RC	80.74%	65.36%	73.53%	69.20%

We achieved an f-measure of 69.20%, which is compatible with the previous state-of-art performance of 67% (Liu et al. 2013) achieved in the diabetes research. The improved precision from combining relation detection with relation classification lies in the fact that the introduction of relation detection eliminates or at least decreases the influence of drug and event pairs that have no relation. The relatively lower precision is due to the influence of the relation type 'others,' which our rule fails to extract. For example, the following sentence in post 15628 cannot be detected by our rule, so is categorized to 'Adverse Drug Event' by mistake: "Metoprolol is beta blocker; this drug blocks the B1 receptors in heart so if abrupt withdrawal occurs then it can result in to arrhythmia, so ideally it should be withdrawn slowly." The relationship type between the drug "beta blocker" and "arrhythmia" should be 'others.'

In without report source classification (Without RSC), we regard all the sentences as a patient's own experience. To conduct report source classification (RSC), we manually annotated 250 of the 12,976 sentences. One hundred and sixty sentences are from patients' own experiences and 90 sentences are from hearsay. Five-fold cross validation was performed in order to decrease the influence of variability in the training set. As shown in Table 7, the f-measure improved from 69.05% to 90.53% after conducting report source classification.

Table 7. Performance Comparison between RSC and without RSC

Method	Precision	Recall	F-measure
Without RSC	52.73%	100 %	69.05%
RSC	89.65%	91.42%	90.53%

In order to ensure that the assessment does not happen by chance, we conducted pair wise single-sided t tests on f-measure. The p-values for the hypotheses testing for adverse drug event extraction and report source classification are presented in Table 8.

Table 8. P values for adverse drug event extraction and report source classification

Hypothesis No.	Hypothesis	P value for f-measure
1a	RC>CO	0.02299*
1b	RD+RC>RC	0.02565*
2	RSC> without RSC	0.000000657*

Note: Significance level *a=0.05.

The three hypotheses are all supported with p values for f-measure of less than 0.05, indicating the improvement in overall performance is significant.

5   Discussions

We applied information extraction techniques to the entire forum. A summary of the extracted results is shown in Figure 1. There are 18,865 drug-event pairs that co-occur in sentences. Based on our extraction techniques, 6,388 pairs are adverse drug events. Among them, 3,580 pairs are from patients' experience.

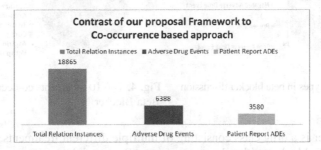

Fig. 1. A summary of extracted patient-reported adverse drug events

Based on the results, we can see that there are a large number of false positive adverse drug events which couldn't be filtered out by the co-occurrence-based approach. Only 33.86% of all the relation instances contain adverse drug events. About 56.04% of these come from patient reports. Only about 18.98% of all relation instances contain adverse drug events that come from patient reports.

We compared the results of our system with FAERS to verify its usefulness. The time span of the forum discussions is January 1995 to January 2014 and that of FAERS is January 2004 to March 2013, the latest released FDA data. The drugs that are usually discussed in the forums differ from those reported to FAERS. In Figure 2, we show the top 10 most discussed treatments from both data sources. Only three drugs overlap.

Beta blocker, calcium channel blocker and statin represent heart disease drug classes instead of an individual drug. This finding indicates that heart disease patients prefer to use general drug classes instead of specific drug names in treatment discussion. There might be a significant number of expert patients who have knowledge about drug classes and their impact in the forum.

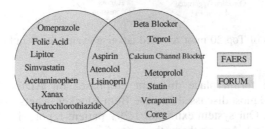

Fig. 2. A comparison of Top 10 most discussed drugs from FAERS and Forum

Beta blocker is the most discussed treatment in the heart disease forum. There are 1,822 discussions about beta blocker and its related medical events. Among them, 71% of them are adverse drug events, 19% are drug indications, 9% are negated adverse drug events and 1% are prevention. A distribution of relation types for extracted beta blocker reports is shown in Figure 3 below.

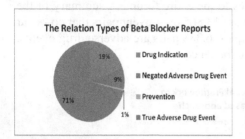

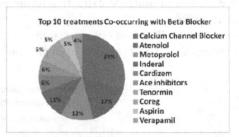

Fig. 3. Relation types in beta blocker discussion   **Fig. 4.** Top 10 treatments co-occurring with Beta Blocker

Beta blocker is a drug class consisting of multiple different treatments. Users often mentioned beta blocker with other treatments. Some of these treatments belong to the same drug class, others are co-medications. Figure 4 shows the top 10 medications co-occurring with beta blocker in the heart disease forum.

Among the top 10 co-occurred treatments, Atenolol, Metoprolol, Tenormin, Coreg and Inderal are beta blocker drugs. Ace inhibitor and calcium channel blocker are drug classes often used along with beta blocker to treat heart disease. Aspirin and Verapamil are not beta blocker treatments. Based on the analysis, we find that 50% of the adverse events related to beta blocker have other co-medications, presenting great potential for identifying drug interactions from these discussions.

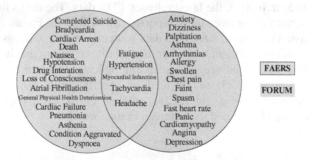

Fig. 5. A comparison of Top 20 most reported adverse events for Beta blocker from FAERS and Forum

FAERS and the forum place different emphases on ADEs. In Figure 5, we compared the top 20 most discussed adverse Beta Blocker events from the forum with those from FAERS. Our system extracted 1,297 patient-reported beta blocker ADEs; FAERS reported 3,162. Among them, there are 5 common ADEs. FAERS focuses on severe ADEs, such as "loss of consciousness" and "death," while forum reports concentrated on mild ADEs such as "anxiety" and "dizziness." Forums seem to be more symptom derived describers while FAERS seems to be more diagnosis derived describers. "Palpitations", "fast heart rate" and "arrhythmia" from forum discussions might be described as atrial fibrillation by the healthcare professionals.

There are several common ADEs between FAERS and our system. Figure 6 shows the top 10 reported adverse events of Beta blocker in the patient forum with the corresponding report number from FAERS. Nine of the top 10 reported adverse events are captured by FAERS. "Arrythmias" does not appear in the FAERS reports. This shows that health social media adverse drug event reports can not only capture well-established adverse event signals but also identify new signals not captured by FAERS. Thus, health social media can be a valuable supplemental data source for drug safety surveillance.

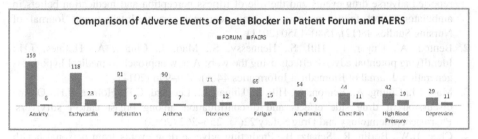

Fig. 6. Comparison of Adverse Beta Blocker Events in Patient Forum and FAERS

6   Conclusion

In light of the need to mine social media for heart disease-related adverse drug events, we developed an information extraction system to identify patient-reported adverse drug events from major health discussion forums. A series of experiments were conducted on a test bed encompassing about 250,000 posts from heart disease forums. The results revealed that our system can effectively extract patient-reported adverse drug events with high performance. This information extraction was based on the framework developed in our previous work on diabetes forums [8]. We demonstrated the generalizability of this approach on different disease discussion forums.

Based on the analysis of extracted adverse drug events from the heart disease forum, we learned that health social media provides information about adverse drug events that are not captured by the FDA's Adverse Event Reporting System. Health social media adverse drug event reports also show great potential to help identify drug interactions for heart disease treatment. Adverse drug event reports from health social media are not biased to severe adverse events as FAERS is. Most of the reports are minor and common adverse events while FAERS has a larger number of severe adverse events. Common and minor side effects that affect quality of life like fatigue, decreased libido, erectile dysfunction, depression can lead to drug non-compliance, a major obstacle of successful treatments. Patients' reporting of these ADEs may explain treatment failures due to non-compliance and would be of interest to treating clinicians and pharmaceutical companies. Patient social media includes treatment experiences from both novice patients and expert patients. The collective patient intelligence on social media has potential to educate more patients about drug safety and treatment management if presented properly and effectively.

Acknowledgement. This work was supported in part by DTRA, #HDTRA1-09-1-0058. We appreciate the contribution of Randall Brown, MD, a physician at University Medical Center University of Arizona, to this study and the research assistance provided by fellow members in the University of Arizona's Artificial Intelligence Lab.

References

1. De Smedt, R.H., Denig, P., van der Meer, K., Haaijer-Ruskamp, F.M., Jaarsma, T.: Self-reported adverse drug events and the role of illness perception and medication beliefs in ambulatory heart failure patients: A cross-sectional survey. International Journal of Nursing Studies 48(12), 1540–1550 (2011)
2. Benton, A., Ungar, L., Hill, S., Hennessy, S., Mao, J., Chung, A., Holmes, J.H.: Identifying potential adverse effects using the web: A new approach to medical hypothesis generation. Journal of Biomedical Informatics 44(6), 989–996 (2011)
3. Mao, J.J., Chung, A., Benton, A., Hill, S., Ungar, L., Leonard, C.E., Holmes, J.H.: Online discussion of drug side effects and discontinuation among breast cancer survivors. Pharmacoepidemiology and Drug Safety 22(3), 256–262 (2013)
4. Chee, B.W., Berlin, R., Schatz, B.: Predicting adverse drug events from personal health messages. In: AMIA Annual Symposium Proceedings, vol. 2011, pp. 217–226 (2011)
5. Leaman, R., Wojtulewicz, L., Sullivan, R., et al.: Towards internet-age pharmacovigilance: extracting adverse drug reactions from user posts to health-related social networks. In: Proceedings of the 2010 Workshop on Biomedical Natural Language Processing, pp. 117–125. Association for Computational Linguistics (2010)
6. Nikfarjam, A., Gonzalez, G.H.: Pattern mining for extraction of mentions of Adverse Drug Reaction from user comments. In: Proceeding of 2011 AMIA Annual Symposium, pp. 1019–1026 (2011)
7. Yang, C., Yang, H., Jiang, L., et al.: Social media mining for drug safety signal detection. In: Proceedings of the 2012 International Workshop on Smart Health and Wellbeing, pp. 33–40. ACM (2012)
8. Liu, X., Chen, H.: AZDrugMiner: an information extraction system for mining patient-reported adverse drug events in online patient forums. In: Zeng, D., Yang, C.C., Tseng, V.S., Xing, C., Chen, H., Wang, F.-Y., Zheng, X. (eds.) ICSH 2013. LNCS, vol. 8040, pp. 134–150. Springer, Heidelberg (2013)
9. Bian, J., Topaloglu, U., Yu, F.: Towards large-scale twitter mining for drug-related adverse events. In: Proceedings of the 2012 International Workshop on Smart Health and Wellbeing, pp. 25–32. ACM (October 2012)
10. MetaMap, http://metamap.nlm.nih.gov
11. Bunescu, R.C., Mooney, R.J.: A shortest path dependency kernel for relation extraction. In: Proceedings of the conference on Human Language Technology and Empirical Methods in Natural Language Processing, pp. 724–731. Association for Computational Linguistics (2005)
12. SVM-light, http://svmlight.joachims.org
13. NegEx, https://code.google.com/p/negex

An Empirical Analysis on Communications about Electronic Nicotine Delivery Systems (ENDS) in Chinese Social Media

Kainan Cui[1,2], Xiaolong Zheng[2], Daniel Zeng[2], and Scott Leischow[3]

[1] The School of Electronic and Information Engineering,
Xi'an Jiaotong University, Xi'an, China
[2] State Key Laboratory of Management and Control for Complex Systems,
Institute of Automation, Chinese Academy of Sciences, Beijing, China
[3] Mayo Clinic in Arizona, Phoenix, USA
kainan.cui@live.cn, xiaolong.zheng@ia.ac.cn

Abstract. China, with a smoking population of over 350 million, is the largest potential market for electronic nicotine delivery systems (ENDS). The importance of understanding how ENDS are promoted and discussed in China cannot be overstated. However, related research is sparse. This study aims to explore the nature and extent of discussions around ENDS in Chinese social media, which have the power to influence a massive audience. We collected the data from Sina Weibo, which is one of the most popular Chinese microblogging sites. The dataset, which consisted of 999 messages, was analyzed in terms of polarities, genres and discussion topics. Statistical test and regression analysis were used to explore whether those features of messages will affect the message popularity, which was measured by repost number and comment number. The results of our study showed that 1) The majority of the messages were Pro-ENDS; 2) The number of comments received by messages of different genes varies significantly; 3) Whether a message contains specific topics or not will affect the comment number.

Keywords: Electronic nicotine delivery devices, public opinion, advertising and Promotion, social media, micro-blogging systems.

1   Introduction

Electronic nicotine delivery systems (ENDS) are battery operated products designed to deliver nicotine by heating nicotine rather than by burning tobacco. Recent years have witnessed tremendous growth in the marketplace of ENDS. China, with a smoking population of over 350 million, is not only the inventor and main provider of ENDS, but also the world's largest potential market for ENDS. Although the market of ENDS in China is still in its infancy, the significance of ENDS on China's tobacco control cannot be overstated.

As inappropriate health claims of ENDS (e.g., ENDS are totally harmless) could misled the public and make damages to the public health [1], such as the marketing

X. Zheng et al. (Eds.): ICSH 2014, LNCS 8549, pp. 37–43, 2014.
© Springer International Publishing Switzerland 2014

campaigns targeted to non-tobacco users, especially young people, have raised great public health concerns over nicotine addiction [2] [3] [4], the empirical analysis to understanding how ENDS are promoted and discussed in China and their impact on general public's attentions and perceptions of ENDS is critically needed. With the rapid growing of social media, there were increasing numbers of studies analyzing the content regarding ENDS in western social media sites, e.g. YouTube[5], Twitter [6] and so on. However, related research is sparse in China.

To fill this important research gap and provide implications for ENDS related policy making in China, we conducted a content analysis on one of the most popular Chinese microblogging sites called Sina Weibo. The main purpose of carrying out this study is twofold: 1) understand the polarities, genres and topics of messages about ENDS in Chinese microblogging sites; 2) understand which factors will affect the social media user's attention on messages about ENDS.

The rest of this paper is organized as follows. In Section 2, we begin with a brief introduction to the dataset and methods we used in this study. We report our empirical analysis results and statistical results in Section 3. We conclude our paper by summarizing the findings and discussing several key issues in Section 4.

2   Methods

In 27 April, 2013 , We collected 2101 raw messages by submitting the Chinese keyword "电子烟" (English: electronic cigarettes) to the official search engine on Sina Weibo. After refining our sample, 999 messages were left in our sample dataset.

To gain understanding of the polarity and gene of ENDS messages, a team of two graduate students with extensive social media analytics and public health informatics training coded the messages independently. The kappa statistics were calculated to test the inter-coder reliability [7]. The team first classified these messages into pro-ENDS, anti-ENDS or "neutral". This polarity code scheme is adapted from[14]. We extended the scheme, which was to code videos regarding little cigars/cigarillos, to the context of ENDS discussion. Pro-ENDS was defined as messages that promoted the use of ENDS. Anti-ENDS was defined as messages that expressed negative attitudes towards ENDS and ENDS promotion. Any messages that were not easily classified as either pro-ENDS or anti-ENDS, but included mention about ENDS, were coded as "neutral".

Messages were also classified into the following genres: "advertisements", "consumer's sharing", "news" and "general discussions" by the same set of coders. The Genres were determined based on the recurring themes of current dataset. "Advertisements" refers to messages that promoted a product or service with commercial purposes. "Consumer's sharing" refers to postings that clearly indicated the poster's personal usage and purchase of ENDS. "News" refers to media reports, which usually consists of a news headline and summary. Some messages also contain links to full story. "General discussions" refers to the rest of messages related to ENDS. The kappa value was 0.92 for coding the polarity of messages and 0.95 for coding the genre of messages which indicate high reliability.

To gain more understanding of the topics discussed in the messages, we developed an issue list based on the recurring themes of current dataset and the previous study about debate of ENDS [8] [9]. There were not only pro-ENDS themes, but also anti-ENDS themes and questions around ENDS. Specifically, the pro-ENDS themes include 1) ENDS are effective to quit smoking, 2) ENDS have health benefits, 3) ENDS are legal to advertise and use, 4) ENDS taste good, 5) ENDS are cheap, 6) ENDS are suitable gifts 7) ENDS have candy flavor. The anti-ENDS themes include 1) ENDS are ineffective to quit smoking, 2) ENDS pose health hazards, 3) ENDS are illegal to advertise and use, 4) ENDS taste bad, 5) ENDS are expensive. The questions of ENDS include 1) Are ENDS effective to quit smoking? 2) Are ENDS healthy? 3) Are ENDS legal? 4) What are ENDS? 5) Where to buy ENDS? 6) Other questions.

In order to compare the popularity of these messages, we performed several statistical tests to assess the distribution of repost number and comment number. In particular, Kruskal-Wallis Test [10] and Mann-Whitney U test [11] were used to analyses differences of message popularity between groups, p values <0.05 were considered statistically significant. Logistic regression was used to assess whether topic contained in messages will affect the message popularity.

3   Results

Among the 999 messages in our sample, 677 messages were pro-ENDS, whereas 164 were anti-ENDS and 158 were "neutral" messages as shown in Table 1. Regarding the statistics associated with messages, pro-ENDS messages received 941 reposts and 1863 comments, which far exceed the corresponding numbers of anti-ENDS and "neutral" messages. Anti-ENDS messages received 221 reposts and 439 comments, "neutral" messages received 375 reposts and 459 comments.

Regarding the gene of messages, 256 messages were coded as "advertisements", which received 286 reposts and 187 comments as shown in Table 1. 244 messages were coded as "consumers' sharing", which received 220 reposts and 1390 comments. 127 messages were coded as "news", which received 451 reposts and 187 comments. The rest messages were coded as "general discussions", which had 372 messages and received 580 reposts and 997 comments.

Table 1. Statistics of messages regarding ENDS by polarities and genes

	# of messages	# of reposts	# of comments
Polarity			
Pro-ENDS messages	677	941	1863
Anti-ENDS messages	164	221	439
"Neutral" messages	158	375	459
Gene			
Advertisements	256	286	187
Consumers' sharing	244	220	1390
News	127	451	187
General discussions	372	580	997

Table 2 presents the statistics of topics discussed in the sample. The most mentioned topic was "ENDS are effective to quit smoking", which had 218 messages and received 223 reposts and 738 comments. The topic receiving most reposts was the health benefits of ENDS, which had 264 reposts.

Table 2. Statistics of discussed topics about ENDS

	# of messages	# of reposts	# of comments
Effectiveness to quit smoking			
Effective	218	223	738
Ineffective	29	107	164
Are ENDS effective?	16	8	86
Health effects of ENDS			
Health benefits	105	264	214
Health hazards	33	27	98
Are ENDS healthy?	7	4	18
Legality of ENDS			
Legal	31	17	76
Illegal	81	71	73
Are ENDS legal?	3	0	16
Taste of ENDS			
Taste good	25	9	73
Taste bad	23	3	119
Price of ENDS			
Cheap	8	11	11
Expensive	6	7	13
Others			
As gifts	78	166	323
Candy flavor	39	20	155
What is ENDS?	11	1	51
Where to buy ENDS?	9	5	50
Other questions	35	4	128

To assess whether the polarity and gene of messages will affect the popularity of messages, we provide the statistical results comparing the mean of messages' comment number and repost number. The Kruskal-Wallis test results indicate that there was no significant difference in comment number, repost number among messages of different polarities. The results of Mann-Whitney U test show that the comment number of anti-ENDS messages and "neutral" messages are no identical (p-value = 0.02898, Mann-Whitney U test), all of other pairs of comparisons are identical.

When it comes to the gene of messages, the mean comment number among "advertisement" messages, "consumers' share" messages, "news" messages and "general discussion messages" were significantly different (p-value < 2.2e-16, Kruskal-Wallis test). As shown in Fig. 1, the slopes of the best fit line among genes vary significantly. The slope of "consumers' share" messages was 5.7 whereas the slope of "advertisement" messages was 0.73. More specially, the mean comment number of "consumers' share" messages was significantly different with "advertisement" messages (p-value < 2.2e-16, Mann-Whitney U), "news" messages (p-value < 2.2e-16, Mann-Whitney U) and "general discussion" messages (p-value = 2.687e-13, Mann-Whitney U). The mean comment number of both "advertisement messages and "news" messages were significantly different with "general discussion" messages. We did not observed significant difference in repost number among messages of different genes.

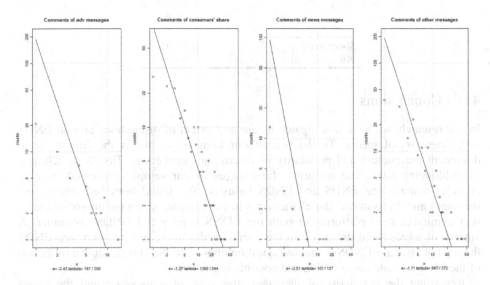

Fig. 1. The comment number distribution of messages by different genes

To investigate the impact of topics discussed in messages on the message popularity, we performed two linear regression analyses. The first regression model included all of the topics which were treated as binary variables. After performing the first analysis, we advanced the regression model by dropping those topic variables whose coefficient was not significant in the first model. The second regression included three topic variables as shown in Formula 1.

$$y = \beta_0 + \beta_1 pt_3 + \beta_2 at_2 + \beta_3 at_3 + \varepsilon \tag{1}$$

Regression analysis results showed that the pt_3 ("ENDS are suitable gifts"), at_2 ("ENDS are ineffective to quit smoking") and at_3 ("ENDS are Illegal") contributed significantly to the prediction of comment number as shown in Table 3. Among the three topics, "ENDS are suitable gifts" and "ENDS are ineffective to quit smoking" will arise more comments whereas "ENDS are illegal" will suppress the discussions.

Table 3. Regression analysis results of using topic predict comment number

	# of messages
Constant	2.7139***
	(0.2081)
Pt_3	1.4271*
	(0.7024)
At_2	2.9412**
	(1.1198)
At_3	-1.8127**
	(0.6805)
R-squared	0.01891
No. observation	999

4   Conclusions

In our research, we have investigated nature and extent of discussions around ENDS in Chinese social media. To the best of our knowledge, this is the first study to document the content and popularity of discussions concerning ENDS on Chinese microblogging sites. The majority of messages in our sample expressed positive attitudes towards the ENDS and ENDS industry. We found both "advertisement" messages and "consumers' share" messages in our sample, which means social media is a communication platform for both the EDNS vendor and ENDS consumer. A variety of topics were discussed in the social media, there are not only pro-ENDS theme, but also anti-ENDS theme and question about ENDS. This result is a reflection of the heated debate about ENDS and possible regulations.

Regarding the popularity of messages, the gene of a message and the topics discussed in a message only influenced the comment number. The polarity of messages affected neither the comment number nor the repost number. "Consumer's share" messages received the most comments while "advertisement" messages received the least comments. This could be explained by the fact that "consumer's share" messages are usually more credible than "advertisement" messages. Social media users are more likely to interact with the users who share their own experience.

One of the limitations in this study is that microblogging is dynamic by nature [12][13]. The message stream changes rapidly, which may affect the representativeness of sample. We need to further analyze and monitor the discussions regarding ENDS to validate our findings. Further, although our dataset was collected from one of the most popular social media websites in China, it is likely that the sample was not representative of ENDS messages in other social media services. It would be beneficial to conduct further research that expands the scope of this analysis to additional social media websites in China.

Acknowledgments. The authors would like to thank Chuan Luo, Saike He, Zhu Zhang for their helpful suggestions. This work was supported in part by the following grants: The National Natural Science Foundation of China, Grant No. 71103180, 91124001, 71025001, and 91024030, by the Early Career Development Award of SKLMCCS and by the Ministry of Health under Grant No. 2012ZX10004801.

References

[1] Benowitz, N.L., Goniewicz, M.L.: The regulatory challenge of electronic cigarettes. JAMA 310, 685–686 (2013)

[2] Pepper, J.K., Reiter, P.L., McRee, A.-L., Cameron, L.D., Gilkey, M.B., Brewer, N.T.: Adolescent Males' Awareness of and Willingness to Try Electronic Cigarettes. J. Adolesc. Health 52, 144–150 (2013)

[3] Lee, S., Kimm, H., Yun, J.E., Jee, S.H.: Public health challenges of electronic cigarettes in South Korea. J. Prev. Med. Public Health 44, 235–241 (2011)

[4] Riker, C.A., Lee, K., Darville, A., Hahn, E.J.: E-Cigarettes: Promise or Peril? Nurs. Clin. North Am. 47, 159–171 (2012)

[5] Bromberg, J.E., Augustson, E.M., Backinger, C.L.: Portrayal of Smokeless Tobacco in YouTube Videos. Nicotine Tob. Res. 14, 455–462 (2012)

[6] Prochaska, J.J., Pechmann, C., Kim, R., Leonhardt, J.M.: Twitter=quitter? An analysis of Twitter quit smoking social networks. Tob. Control 21, 447–449 (2012)

[7] Carletta, J.: Assessing agreement on classification tasks: the kappa statistic. Comput. Linguist. 22, 249–254 (1996)

[8] Henningfield, J.E., Zaatari, G.S.: Electronic nicotine delivery systems: emerging science foundation for policy. Tob. Control 19, 89–90 (2010)

[9] de Andrade, M., Hastings, G.: The marketing of e-cigarettes: a UK snapshot (2013), http://blogs.bmj.com/tc/2013/04/06/the-marketing-of-e-cigarettes-a-uk-snapshot/ (accessed: July 22, 2013)

[10] McKight, P.E., Najab, J.: Kruskal-Wallis Test. In: The Corsini Encyclopedia of Psychology. John Wiley & Sons, Inc. (2010)

[11] Mann–Whitney U, Wikipedia, the free encyclopedia (April 30, 2014)

[12] Freeman, B.: New media and tobacco control. Tob. Control 21, 139–144 (2012)

[13] Zeng, D., Chen, H., Lusch, R., Li, S.-H.: Social Media Analytics and Intelligence. Intell. Syst. IEEE 25, 13–16 (2010)

Analyzing Spatio-temporal Patterns of Online Public Attentions in Emergency Events: A Case Study of 2009 H1N1 Influenza Outbreak in China

Kainan Cui[1,2], Xiaolong Zheng[2], Zhu Zhang[2], and Daniel Zeng[2]

[1] The School of Electronic and Information Engineering,
Xi'an Jiaotong University, Xi'an, China
[2] State Key Laboratory of Management and Control for Complex Systems,
Institute of Automation, Chinese Academy of Sciences, Beijing, China
kainan.cui@live.cn, xiaolong.zheng@ia.ac.cn

Abstract. Understanding the public attention and perception towards epidemics is critical for public health response. However, the research question concerning the spatio-temporal patterns of public attention and the interactions with media attention and severity of epidemic is still not well studied. Aim to fill this research gap, we chose the H1N1 influenza outbreak in the mainland of China in 2009 as case to study the spatio-temporal patterns of public attention, and their correlations with media attention and severity of epidemic. The results of this paper indicate that public attention and media attention had high correlation from both temporal and spatial perspectives, which can provide us significant insights to understand the collective behavior of massive online users during emergency events.

Keywords: Information diffusion, public attenion, emergency response, influenza, epidemic outbreaks.

1 Introduction

The development of crisis situations was significantly affected by the rapid diffusion of information and opinions through Internet[1][2][3][4][5]. As recent studies suggested that the general public's attention and perception regarding epidemics also plays important role in the evolution process of epidemics[6], studying temporal and geospatial patterns of online public attention can uncover useful mechanism of information diffusion during emergency event to facilitate public health response and possibly prevention measures.

Many researches show that open source information has great application potential for improving the situational awareness during emergency situation. There are already lots of attempts and applications using different online data, such as search engine logs[7][8][9], news[10][11], blogs [12], micro-blog [13] and wiki [14], to predict the number of infections, track the transmission rate and study the response behavior for influenza outbreak. However, the question concerning the temporal and spatial

X. Zheng et al. (Eds.): ICSH 2014, LNCS 8549, pp. 44–50, 2014.

patterns of public attention and the interaction with media attention and severity of epidemic remain largely unexplored.

In order to fill this important research gap and provide implications for decision making during emergency, we chose the H1N1 influenza outbreak in the mainland of China in 2009 as case in this paper. In particular, we performed time series analysis on the online news and corresponding comments at first. Then we performed spatial analysis to study the spatial pattern and evolution process. Our results indicate that public attention towards emergency event had high correlation and similar temporal, geospatial patterns with media attention. The correlation between public attention and severity of epidemic was not stable which needs further study.

The rest of this paper is organized as follows. In Section 2, we begin with a brief introduction to the dataset we used in this study. We report our empirical analysis result and statistical results in Section 3. We conclude our paper by summarizing the findings and discussing several key issues in Section 4.

2   Data and Methods

2.1   Dataset

We chose the H1N1 influenza outbreak in the mainland of China in 2009 as the case to study the public attention during emergency events. Our dataset is composed by three parts, which are news data, comment data and epidemic data. We obtained news data (referred as SINA-ND) and comment data (referred as SINA-CD) from Sina news (news.sina.com), which is a famous online media offering a full array of Chinese-language reports and information.

Sina news provided a special repost regarding H1N1 outbreak, which is available at http://news.sina.com.cn/z/zhuliugan/index.shtml. We developed a customized crawler for collecting data. After removing duplicated data, there are 3303 news covering the period from April 26, 2009 to August 10 2010 and 75878 comments covering the period from May 27, 2009 to August 11, 2010.

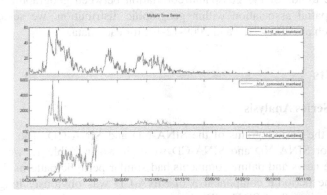

Fig. 1. The comment number distribution of messages by different genes

The epidemic data (referred as CH-ED) used in our study is obtained through an authority website, which serves 31 province-level regions in the mainland of China and covers the period from May 11, 2009 to July 9, 2009. Fig. 1 shows the time series plot of SINA-ND, SINA-CD and CH-ED.

2.2   Time Series Analysis Methods

Periodogram [15] (also known as spectral plot) is applied to assess the periodicity of online news and corresponding comments. A peak in the periodogram indicates there is a periodic component near the value corresponding to the peak. To extract the amplitude of a periodic component data, ideal pass filter is applied for the periodogram to filter the raw data, with the frequency interval covering the peak shape in the periodogramls.

To examine the associations between time series of news and comments, news and cases, comments and cases, cross-correlation is used to measure the degree of the linear relationship between two time series with limited time lags (ten days in this study). A specific lag corresponding to a high correlation of two time series may indicate that these two series have certain same influencing factors and a time delay.

2.3   Geospatial Analysis Methods

We chose the Pearson's correlation coefficient to measure the spatial correlation between two geographic distributions. In particular, we computed the correlation value of SINA-ND and SINA-CD, SINA-ND and CH-ED, SINA-CD and CH-ED respectively. We defined P < 0.01 as statistically significant. After the correlation analyses, several geospatial distribution plots were generated for visual comparison on geospatial patterns.

Global Moran's I[16][17]   is selected to quantify the geospatial correlation within one geographic distribution. In particular, we computed the association value of SINA-ND, SINA-CD and CH-ED respectively. In order to gain more understanding of the change trends of the geospatial correlation between geographic distributions and the geospatial association within geographic distribution, we select two time snapshot, which are 2009-7-19 and 2009-12-12, for each data.

3   Results

3.1   Time Series Analysis

Fig. 2 shows the periodograms of the SINA-ND and SINA-CD. The main periodic components for SINA-ND and SINA-CD were shown in Table 1., we can observe that the online news and online comments had similar periodic patterns. In particular, except that the periodic component 3 of SINA-CD was obviously longer than the periodic component 3 of SINA-ND, the rest periodic components of SINA-CD and corresponding periodic components of SINA-ND had almost the same period length.

Regarding the amplitude of periodic component, the comments were greater than the news, which means the daily post number of comments is more volatile than daily post number of news,

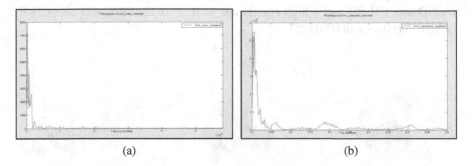

(a)   (b)

Fig. 2. The periodograms of the time series of SINA-ND (a) and SINA-CD (b)

Table 1. A comparison of periodic components for SINA-ND and SINA-CD

	Salient peak	Period(day)	Amplitude
SINA-ND (news)			
periodic component 1	0.002123	471.0094	16
periodic component 2	0.00637	156.9859	12
periodic component 3	0.0127	78.74016	10
periodic component 4	0.0212	47.16981	4
SINA-CD (comments)			
periodic component 1	0.002118	472.1435	440
periodic component 2	0.006356	157.3341	420
periodic component 3	0.0106	94.33962	320
periodic component 4	0.0212	47.16981	200

The correlation results and the corresponding time lag were shown in Table 2. These lags are selected to provide the highest correlation for each pair. From Table 2, we can observe significant positive correlation between the news and comments. The correlation degree between news and cases was larger than comments and cases.

Table 2. Cross-correlation results among SINA-ND, SINA-CD and CH-ED

	Time lag	Highest correlation
SINA-ND and CH-ED	-10	0.21
SINA-ND and SINA-CD	-1	0.715
SINA-CD and CH-ED	-10	0.125

3.2   Geospatial Analysis

Fig. 3 shows that the three datasets have a similar geospatial distribution. From a qualitative perspective, SINA-ND and SIND-CD had a high correlation of 0.9488, SINA-ND and CH-ED had a high correlation of 0. 872672; SINC-CD and CH-ED had a high correlation of 0.805023.

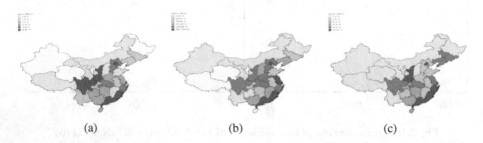

(a)   (b)   (c)

Fig. 3. Geospatial distribution before July 192, 2009 of SINA-ND (a), SIND-CD (b) and CH-ED (c)

Fig. 4 shows that the SINA-ND and SINA-CD had a similar geospatial distribution. From a qualitative perspective, SINA-ND and SIND-CD had a high correlation of 0.962354 while SINA-ND and CH-ED had a low correlation of 0.1870, SINC-CD and CH-ED had a low correlation of 0.3363.

The statistics of global Moran's I are summarized in Table 3. From this table, we obtain the following observations 1) the offline data (CH-ED-0719 and CH-ED-1222) had higher geospatial association than online data (SINA-ND and SINA-CD) 2) the geospatial association degree for both offline data and online increased over time. 3) The geospatial association degree of online data grew faster than offline data.

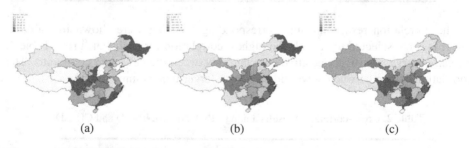

(a)   (b)   (c)

Fig. 4. Geospatial distribution before December 12, 2009 of SINA-ND (a), SIND-CD (b) and CHINA-ED (c)

Table 3. A comparison for the geospatial association of SINA-ND, SINA-CD and CH-ED in different time snapshot

	Moran's I	999 MC simulation		
		E(i)	S_d	Z-score
SINA-ND-0719	0.279	-0.0323	0.826	0.3236
SINA-CD-0719	0.125	-0.0323	0.0863	1.0613
CH-ED-0719	0.439	-0.0323	0.0933	0.0436
SINA-ND-1222	0.313	-0.0323	0.0767	-0.527
SINA-CD-1222	0.421	-0.0323	0.0927	-0.2845
CH-ED-1222	0.444	-0.0323	0.1059	0.0327

4   Conclusions

In this paper we attempt to show the patterns of public attention during epidemic outbreaks from both temporal and spatial perspectives. In particular, we chose H1N1 outbreaks in China mainland as case to examine the periodicity pattern and geospatial association of the media attention (online news) and the public attention (online comments). We also provided temporal and spatial correlation analysis results among media attention, public attention and severity of epidemic.

The results of this study show that the public attention and the media attention had high correlation from both temporal and spatial perspectives, which was agreed with the agenda setting theory. Furthermore the public attention has similar periodicity pattern with media attention, and swung more drastic. This phenomenon could be explained by the herd behavior.

We did not observe stable geospatial correlation between the severity of epidemic and the public attention. The geospatial association of public attention and media attention had increased over time. Further investigation is needed to uncover the mechanism under these empirical results.

One of the limitations in this study is that H1N1 is a brand-new disease affecting the globe which arise great attention from both online media and Web users. However for other diseases or events which Web users concerned not very much, the patterns and features of public attention may vary significantly. However, this work still shed light on the temporal and spatial patterns of public attention during emergency events. Further empirical work is needed to verify our findings.

Acknowledgments. The authors would like to thank Zhidong Cao, Saike He, Chuan Luo for their helpful suggestions. This work was supported in part by the following grants: The National Natural Science Foundation of China, Grant No. 71103180, 91124001, 71025001,and 91024030, by the Early Career Development Award of SKLMCCS and by the Ministry of Health under Grant No. 2012ZX10004801.

References

[1] Zeng, D., Chen, H., Lusch, R., Li, S.-H.: Social Media Analytics and Intelligence. Intell.Syst. IEEE 25, 13–16 (2010)

[2] Zheng, X., Zhong, Y., Zeng, D., Wang, F.-Y.: Social influence and spread dynamics in social networks. Front. Comput. Sci. 6(5), 611–620 (2012)

[3] Wang, Y., Zeng, D., Zheng, X., Wang, F.: Propagation of online news: Dynamic patterns. In: IEEE International Conference on Intelligence and Security Informatics, ISI 2009, pp. 257–259 (2009)

[4] Wang, Y., Zeng, D., Zhu, B., Zheng, X., Wang, F.: Patterns of news dissemination through online news media: A case study in China. Inf. Syst. Front., 1–14 (July 2012)

[5] Zheng, X., Zeng, D., Wang, F.-Y.: Social balance in signed networks. Inf. Syst. Front., 1–19 (January 2014)

[6] SteelFisher, G.K., Blendon, R.J., Bekheit, M.M., Lubell, K.: The Public's Response to the 2009 H1N1 Influenza Pandemic. N. Engl. J. Med. 362(22), e65 (2010)

[7] Ginsberg, J., Mohebbi, M.H., Patel, R.S., Brammer, L., Smolinski, M.S., Brilliant, L.: Detecting influenza epidemics using search engine query data. Nature 457(7232), 1012–1014 (2009)

[8] Wilson, K., Brownstein, J.S.: Early detection of disease outbreaks using the Internet. Can. Med. Assoc. J. 180(8), 829–831 (2009)

[9] Luo, Y., Zeng, D., Cao, Z., Zheng, X., Wang, Y., Wang, Q., Zhao, H.: Using multi-source web data for epidemic surveillance: A case study of the 2009 Influenza A (H1N1) pandemic in Beijing. In: 2010 IEEE International Conference on Service Operations and Logistics and Informatics (SOLI), pp. 76–81 (2010)

[10] Collier, N., Doan, S., Kawazoe, A., Goodwin, R.M., Conway, M., Tateno, Y., Ngo, Q.-H., Dien, D., Kawtrakul, A., Takeuchi, K., Shigematsu, M., Taniguchi, K.: BioCaster: detecting public health rumors with a Web-based text mining system. Bioinformatics 24(24), 2940–2941 (2008)

[11] Cui, K., Cao, Z., Zheng, X., Zeng, D., Zeng, K., Zheng, M.: A Geospatial Analysis on the Potential Value of News Comments in Infectious Disease Surveillance. In: Chau, M., Wang, G.A., Zheng, X., Chen, H., Zeng, D., Mao, W. (eds.) PAISI 2011. LNCS, vol. 6749, pp. 85–93. Springer, Heidelberg (2011)

[12] Corley, C.D., Cook, D.J., Mikler, A.R., Singh, K.P.: Text and Structural Data Mining of Influenza Mentions in Web and Social Media. Int. J. Environ. Res. Public. Health 7(2), 596–615 (2010)

[13] Culotta, A.: Towards Detecting Influenza Epidemics by Analyzing Twitter Messages. In: Proceedings of the First Workshop on Social Media Analytics, New York, NY, USA, pp. 115–122 (2010)

[14] Laurent, M., Vickers, T.J.: Seeking Health Information Online: Does Wikipedia Matter? J. Am. Med. Inform. Assoc. 16(4), 471–479 (2009)

[15] Zhang, Z., Zheng, X., Zeng, D.D., Cui, K., Luo, C., He, S., Leischow, S.: Discovering seasonal patterns of smoking behavior using online search information. In: 2013 IEEE International Conference on Intelligence and Security Informatics (ISI), pp. 371–373 (2013)

[16] Moran, P.: The Interpretation of Statistical Maps. J. R. Stat. Soc. Ser. B-Stat. Methodol. 10(2), 243–251 (1948)

[17] Cao, Z., Zeng, D., Zheng, X., Wang, Q., Wang, F., Wang, J., Wang, X.: Spatio-temporal evolution of Beijing 2003 SARS epidemic. Sci. China Earth Sci. 53(7), 1017–1028 (2010)

HealthQA: A Chinese QA Summary System for Smart Health

Yanshen Yin[1], Yong Zhang[1], Xiao Liu[2], Yan Zhang[1], Chunxiao Xing[1], and Hsinchun Chen[1,2]

[1] Research Institute of Information Technology,
Tsinghua National Laboratory for Information Science and Technology,
Department of Computer Science and Technology,
Tsinghua University, Beijing, China
[2] Artificial Intelligence Lab, University of Arizona
yys12@mails.tsinghua.edu.cn,
{zhangyong05,xingcx}@tsinghua.edu.cn, xiaoliu@email.arizona.edu,
zhangyan023@gmail.com, hchen@eller.arizona.edu

Abstract. Although online health expert QA services can provide high quality information for health consumers, there is no Chinese question answering system built on knowledge from existing expert answers, leading to duplicated efforts of medical experts and reduced efficiency. To address this issue, we develop a Chinese QA system for smart health (HealthQA), which provides timely, automatic and valuable QA service. Our HealthQA collects diabetes expert question answer data from three major QA websites in China. We develop a hierarchical clustering method to group similar questions and answers, an extended similarity evaluation algorithm for retrieving relevant answers and a ranking based summarization for representing the answer. ROUGE and manual tests show that our system significantly outperforms the search engine.

Keywords: QA system, health, Chinese, summarization, similarity evaluation.

1 Introduction

The increasing prevalence of chronic diseases, such as hypertension, diabetes, heart disease and cancer, as well as the aging problem has resulted in a severe shortage in healthcare resources, including health educators, nurses, physicians, and hospital beds. Consequently, health consumers look for other sources for health information and efficient clinical care. Among the most accessible and cost efficient alternatives are the uses of search engines and question answering services. Search engines are usually general purpose. They retrieve a large number of often redundant and unsynthesized documents in answer to health queries. Online question answering services provide a platform for Internet users to form a social community and exchange knowledge in the form of questions and answers. Generally, there are two types of question answering services: community-based and expert-based. Anyone can ask and answer questions on any topic in community-based question answering

X. Zheng et al. (Eds.): ICSH 2014, LNCS 8549, pp. 51–62, 2014.
© Springer International Publishing Switzerland 2014

services, and people seeking information are connected to those who know the answer. Expert question answering services typically have a large number of information seekers asking questions and a small number of domain experts providing technically correct, complete and reliable answers. Health expert question answering services are highly valued as they satisfy health consumers' demand for high quality information from credible sources and have the potential to empower patients' self-management.

Although online expert QA services can provide high quality health information for health consumers, current practice still has several limitations. Firstly, there are only a small number of qualified (medical) experts to provide answers to many questions, leading to long response time. Secondly, health consumers' questions are colloquial. There might be a significant number of duplicate or similar questions, resulting in repeating efforts from medical experts and reduced efficiency. Thirdly, valuable existing answers haven't been utilized to provide more timely and cost efficient responses to consumers.

To address these issues, we are motivated to develop a heath expert QA summarization system. We aim to summarize reliable expert responses and generate high quality answers based upon health consumers' inquiries. In our health QA summarization system, we develop an advanced similarity evaluation based query component for retrieving relevant questions from existing knowledge bases, a tf-idf based approach to extract the meaningful keywords from the corpus and sentence ranking based summarization for answer representation.

The remainder of the paper is organized as follows. Section 2 provides a review of related work and identifies research gaps. Section 3 describes the HealthQA architecture. Section 4 describes the experiments. Section 5 includes an experimental evaluation of our system. Finally, Section 6 outlines conclusions and future directions.

2   Related Work

2.1   Question Answering System

Question answering is considered an advanced form of information retrieval, which aims to retrieve information in response to users' queries. Many types of QA systems have been developed.

Question answering systems can be categorized into open-domain systems and restricted-domain systems [1]. Open-domain question answering covers a broad range of questions and retrieves information from general ontologies and Internet. The first open-domain question answering system, START, was developed in 1993, and answers general questions based on web data [2]. Other open-domain systems include QuALiM [3] based on Wikipedia data and NSIR [4] and ASU QA [5] based on web data. Restricted-domain question answering systems are built for very specific domains and exploit expert knowledge. Addressing clinical question answering has been an active effort of the biomedical and question answering research community. Cimino et al. [6] developed and evaluated the first medical question answering system (MedQA) based on Medline data. AskHERMES, an online question answering system, was developed based on Medline abstracts, PubMed Central full-text articles and clinical documents for physicians [7]. MiPACQ, a web-based question answering system for clinicians or investigators, integrated multiple NLP tools and machine learning techniques to re-rank answers from medical literature [8]. These systems usually can respond to questions from physicians with high accuracy but require extensive language processing.

Most question answering systems are in English due to the large amount of knowledge and resources available in English. However, several recent studies have investigated QA systems in other languages. Ko et al. [9] developed a multilingual open-domain question answering system for English, Chinese and Japanese. Peng et al. [10] presented a Chinese QA system for a restricted domain. Zhang et al. [11] developed a Chinese QA system for disease inquires.

2.2   Related Techniques

Although there are many variations in QA system architecture for different purposes, there are two major challenges in developing medical QA systems: retrieving documents relevant to the questions and representing answers based on retrieved documents [9]. Document retrieval is an information retrieval task, while answer representation can be considered as text summarization. In order to develop a health-focused question answering system, we focus our survey of literature on these two core techniques applied in prior medical question answering systems.

Information Retrieval

The most commonly adopted approach for information retrieval is vector space model, where documents and queries are represented as vectors of features representing words that occur within the documents [12]. The value of the feature is a function of the term's frequency. Cosine similarity or dot product functions are adopted to compute the similarity between queries and documents.

The vector space model is widely adopted because of its simplicity. However, due to its several obvious drawbacks, various representations have been developed to address these issues such as reducing words to step form [13] and phrases [14]. In addition to improving representation, conceptual and lexical resources, such as Wikipedia [15] and WordNet [17] are brought in to handle words or phrases that are in different forms but share the same meaning.

Besides cosine similarity, many other similarity measures have been developed. Hassan et al. [15] computed the similarity by the sum of the strongest semantic pairings between words. Guo et al. [16] proposed a novel measure that modeled the missing words (words that aren't in the sentence) to tell what the sentence was not about.

To further enhance the retrieval performance, researchers investigated the use of syntactic features in information retrieval. Li et al. [17] proposed a new approach to evaluate and combine the semantic and syntactic similarity (in terms of word order).

In their approaches, two kinds of vectors for each sentence are generated, a semantic vector and an order vector. Order vector indicates the position of each word in a sentence.

Summarization

Summarization aims to generate a document or document set summary. Text summarization can be categorized into single-document summarization and multi-document summarization.

For single-document summarization, Carbonell et al. [18] proposed the Maximal Marginal Relevance (MMR) method to generate a summary. MMR considers both the diversity and relevance of the summary. MMR needs various heuristics to indicate the information quantity. These indicators include tf-idf and sentence keywords. Mittal et al. [19] listed heuristics in three levels: sub-document level, sentence level and word level. These ideas inspire the research on multi-document summarization. To summarize multiple documents, Goldstein et al. [20] extended MMR to MMR-MD by adding cluster and time-sequence components to extract relevant and timely summaries with no redundancy.

In the last decade, many new novel methods have been proposed. Song et al. [21] proposed a method to gauge a word's importance relative to the query. This method categorized the words into three types: query common words, query aspect words and global background words. They utilized composite query to gather additional information specific to the original query and identified query aspect dependent words by comparing the search results of different types of component queries. Some other methods do not operate on word level. Wang et al. [22] developed a sentence-based topic model to detect the latent topic of the sentences in a document and then extracted the top sentences in each topic to form a summary.

2.3   Research Gaps and Questions

After reviewing existing question answering systems, we find that only a few emphasize healthcare. Most medical question answering systems use medical literature as their knowledge bases. None has utilized the expert knowledge publicly available on expert QA websites. Most medical question answering systems are designed for physicians and clinicians. While there is an increasing demand for health information from patients and health consumers, there is no system designed to serve their need. Most medical QA systems are developed in English. Few of them investigated other languages such as Chinese.

In this study, we aim to develop a health QA system that utilizes the medical knowledge from Chinese health expert QA websites and provides accurate and high quality answers for health consumers through summarizing existing answers to similar questions. We propose the following research question: How can we develop a high performance health question answering system that can retrieve relevant questions and existing expert answers based on user queries and summarize answers in an accurate and meaningful manner?

3   Research Design

QA summary system for Health (HealthQA) consists of four major components: health expert QA data collection, expert QA clustering, user query processing and answer summarization.   Figure 1 shows the system architecture.

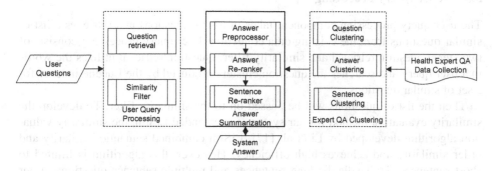

Fig. 1. Research Architecture

3.1   Health Expert QA Data Collection

We investigated most of the known diabetes health QA websites and finally chose three main websites based on their question amount, user activity and answer quality: ask.39.net, club.xywy.com and 120ask.com. We collected all the diabetic QA webpages with an automated web crawler and parsed question title, question content, answer title and answer content from downloaded web pages. For data preprocessing, we adopted the Natural Language Processing and Information Retrieval Sharing System (NLPIR)[1] for word segmentation in Chinese considering its efficiency and accuracy.

3.2   Expert QA Data Clustering

To explore the underlying characteristics of the expert QA dataset and generate relevant answers for summarization, we developed a hierarchical clustering method to group similar questions and answers. Hierarchical clustering usually causes performance issues in large datasets due to computational complexity. To alleviate this, we developed a question clustering method based on Lucene indexing that efficiently clustered all the questions into small groups. We then performed hierarchy clustering algorithm on the small groups. We clustered the answers with the same procedure as well.

After clustering, tf-idf metrics are used to identify keywords to represent each cluster. We treat each cluster as a document and compute the tf-idf for each word.

---

[1] www.nlpir.org/

The words with the top 10% tf-idf scores from each cluster are extracted as keywords to represent the cluster. These keywords are called "question keywords" (QKW) in question clusters and "answer keywords" (AKW) in answer clusters. These keywords will be utilized in the re-ranker to indicate the information quantity.

3.3   User Query Processing

The user query processing component takes in user's questions and retrieves a list of similar questions from the existing data collection. User query processing consists of two steps: question retrieval and similarity filter. Question retrieval utilizes the words in a user query and searches the question clusters produced by the Lucene indexer for a set of similar questions.

Then the list of questions will be passed on to the similarity filter. To develop the similarity evaluation method for our system, we extended LiSim, the similarity valuation algorithm developed by Li et al. [17]. LiSim combined semantic similarity and order similarity and achieves high efficiency. However, this algorithm is limited to short sentences. To handle the long sentences and multiple sentence questions in our corpus, we developed a similarity filter based on the similarity evaluation indicators defined in the equation below.

$$iSim = \sum_{ss_1 \; in \; s_1} \frac{length(ss_1)}{length(s_1)} \cdot LiSim(ss_1, \arg\max_{ss_2 \; in \; s_2} cosine(ss_2, ss_1))$$

s_1 and s_2 are the sentences to compare. For each sub-sentence ss_1 in s_1, calculate the cosine similarity with each sub-sentence ss_2 in s_2. Then choose the most similar sub-sentence in s_2 to calculate the LiSim similarity with ss_1, and then sum all the similarities weighted by $length(ss_1)/length(s_1)$. The weight can automatically weaken the short sub-sentences similarity and strengthen the long sub-sentences similarity, and achieve better internal balance of sentences. Due to the low dimension, cosine similarity calculation is very efficient and has low cost. The main cost is linear to the cost of LiSim, which is efficient too.

3.4   Answer Summarization

Answer summarization consists of three major steps: answer preprocessing, answer re-ranker and sentence re-ranker. Answer Preprocessor first retrieves the similar questions suggested by the user query component and then removes the redundant answers.

Answer Re-ranker evaluates answers (with rank-score) based on a set of answer ranking indicators including tf-idf, question keywords, statistics and question similarity. Each of the indicators is explained in the following table.

Table 1. Answer re-ranker indicators

Indicators	Formula	Definition
Tf-idf	$I_{TFIDF}(a) = \sum_w tfidf_a(w)$	For each answer a, the tf-idf score of a is the sum of the tf-idf scores of all the words in the answer.
Question keyword	$I_{QKW}(a) = \sum_{w \in TopM\_QKW} \alpha_w \cdot tf_a(w)$	For each answer a, the question keyword indicator is the sum of term frequency of keyword w multiplied by the keyword weight (tf-idf score) in the question cluster.
Question Statistics	$I_{STAT}(a) = 2^{\frac{SN_{aver}}{SN(a)}} + 2^{\frac{WN_{aver}}{WN(a)}} + 2^{\frac{CN_{aver}}{CN(a)}}$	For answer a, statistic indicator is the normalized sum of sentence number SN(a), word number WN(a), character number CN(a).
Question similarity	$I_{QUES\_SIM}(a) = Sim(q(a), q_u)$	For answer a, question similarity indicator represents the similarity score between user query and the question leading to answer a.

The tf-idf indicator indicates the uniqueness of a document. The tf-idf score shows the normalized term frequency by inversed document frequency (idf). A low value tf-idf indicates that there's no unique information in the document. The question keyword indicator indicates the information quantity of the answer to the question. When this indicator obtains a high value, the answer covers most keywords for questions similar to the user query. The question statistic indicator indicates the information quantity normalized by answer length. Longer answers tend to carry more information. The statistic indicator balances the answer length and information quantity. The question similarity indicator indicates the relevance of the answer. The more similar to the user's query the question is, the more relevant the question's answer will be. Overall indicator is the sum of the above four indicators.

Sentence Re-ranker evaluates sentences (with rank-score) based on a set of sentence ranking indicators including tf-idf, question keyword indicator, statistic indicator, answer keyword indicator, cluster indicator, position indicator and answer indicator. Each of the indicators is explained in the following table.

Table 2. Sentence re-ranker indicators

Indicators	Formula	Definition
Tf-idf	$I_{TFIDF}(s) = \sum_w tfidf_s(w)$	For sentence s, the tf-idf score is the sum of the tf-idf scores of all the words in the sentence.
Question keyword	$I_{QKW}(s) = \sum_{w \in TopM\_QKW} \alpha_w \cdot tf_s(w)$	For sentence s, the question keyword indicator is the sum of term frequency of keyword w in s multiplied by the keyword weight (tf-idf score) in the question cluster.
Question Statistics	$I_{STAT}(s) = 2^{\frac{WN_{aver}}{WN(s)}} + 2^{\frac{CN_{aver}}{CN(s)}}$	For sentence s, statistic indicator is the normalized sum of word number WN(s) and character number CN(s).
Answer keyword	$I_{AKW}(s) = \sum_{w \in TopM\_AKW} \beta_w \cdot tf_s(w)$	For sentence s, the answer keyword indicator is the sum of term frequency of keyword w in s multiplied by the keyword weight (tf-idf score) in the answer cluster.
Cluster	$I_{CLUSTER}(s) = \frac{\mid C_s \mid}{average \mid C \mid \atop C \in \{all\,C\}}$	For sentence s, the cluster indicator is the number of sentences in the same cluster as s divided by average number of sentences in all the clusters.
Position	$I_{POS}(s) = \frac{SN(a) - p}{SN(a)}$	For sentence s, the position indicator is the number of remaining sentences after sentence s in the answer divided by the number of sentences in the answer.
Answer	$I_{ANS\_SCORE}(s) = I_{overall}(a)$	For sentence s, the answer indictor is the sum of the four answer re-ranking indicators sentence s belongs to.

Answer keyword indicator indicates the information quantity of the sentence. Cluster indicator demonstrates the sizes of the cluster a sentence belongs to. As people usually express important information first in an answer, the position indicator of the sentences can represent the importance of the sentence. Answer score indicator reflects the ranking of the answer a sentence belongs to.

It is important to determine what answers to present to users. The best way to solve the problem is combining the high-rank sentences to form a fluent answer, which is very hard to realize and has been studied for years. The temporary expedient in our research is to show both the highest-rank answer and a few other high-rank sentences to users.

4   Experiment

4.1   Data

Web Crawled Data
Our dataset is from three mainstream health QA websites in China: xywy.com, ask.39.net and 120ask.com. The questions are generated by Chinese users and the answers are published by Chinese doctors. Table 3 demonstrates the data statistics.

Table 3. Dataset description

	Xyxy.com	Ask.39.net	120ask.com	Total
Number of Questions	28,697	73,765	33,247	135,709
Number of Answers	68,497	110,192	71,319	250,008
Time span	2013.4-2013.12	2008.3-2013.12	2012.8-2013.12	

Manually Labeled Data
To evaluate our system, we selected 100 questions, queried our system, and got the relevant questions and all the corresponding answers. Then we provided the questions and answers to four annotators and asked them to write answers for each question (summarize) of 300 words or less. This gave us four different summarized answers for each question, which can reduce the personal bias during summarization. We treated these summaries as the standard answers for our experiment.

4.2   Evaluation Metrics

We performed ROUGE-N, ROUGE-SU and manual testing on our system. ROUGE [23] is an automatic evaluation metric for summarization. It is a set of recall-based metrics measuring the overlapping units between the computer-generated summaries and the ideal summaries created by humans. ROUGE-N is based on N-gram; ROUGE-SU-N is skip-bigram plus unigram-based with a maximum skip distance of N between bigrams. It's widely adopted in many areas.

We also conduct a manual evaluation to compare the informativeness of our summaries with that of the best answers given by a search engine [24]. Best Answers refer to answers ranked first by the search engine. Three annotators are asked to determine whether a summary is better than, equal to or worse than its corresponding best answer in terms of informativeness. Voting strategy is used to determine the final label. If three labels are all different, it is labeled as unknown.

4.3   Evaluation

Generated Answers vs. Search Engine Answer

We compared our generated answer summaries with the first answer from search engine (Lucene) to test whether our approach was valuable.

Table 4 compares our results (denoted as HealthQA) with the search engine's best answer. HealthQA selects the top 300 words generated by our summary system. Evaluation results show that HealthQA outperforms the search engine result. Among these, ROUGE-1 of HealthQA is 36% higher, ROUGE-2 is 38% higher, but ROUGE-SU4 is equal to the search engine. The evaluation scores decrease from ROUGE-1 to ROUGE-SU4, because the standard answers tend to contain more annotators' vocabulary while system outputs reuse the original wording from the answers. ROUGE-1 compares the generated answer to the standard answer in word level without considering the order. HealthQA significantly outperforms search engine in ROUGE-1, indicating the summary produced by HealthQA conveys more information in semantic level than the search engine answer.

The absolute low ROUGE-SU4 is due to the syntactic difference between standard answer and generated answer. Both HealthQA and search engine get the same score in ROUGE-SU4. HealthQA and the search engine achieve similar performance in capturing users' syntactic habits as they both utilize original representations rather than generate new sentences.

Table 4. Comparison of Summarization Performance

Method	ROUGE-1	ROUGE-2	ROUGE-SU4
HealthQA	0.60	0.40	0.26
Search Engine	0.44	0.29	0.26

Manual Evaluation

ROUGE test provides quantitative evidence to verify HealthQA's performance. However, it doesn't reflect the usefulness of the system from users' perspectives. Thus, we conduct a survey from end users to compare the performance of our system to that of the search engine. We randomly find 3 ordinary users with no knowledge about our system, provide them with 100 randomly selected questions and corresponding answers from HealthQA and search engine. They will check the questions, and choose which answer is better or equal than the other answer.

Table 5 shows the users' feedback to both our answers and the best answers given by search engine. We can see from the table that HealthQA receives more than half of the votes and the search engine receives only 8% of votes. In the meanwhile, 37% of the answers are equal between HealthQA and search engine. This result shows that more that 91% of the answers produced by HealthQA are accepted by the users.

Table 5. User's feedback to answers from HealthQA and search engine

Users' Opinion	HealthQA Better	Search Engine Better	Equal	Unknown
Vote	54%	8%	37%	1%

4.4   Sample HealthQA Output

Table 6 gives a sample output of HealthQA. The question is about drugs and therapies for Type II diabetes. HealthQA's answer performs better than the search engine's in terms of information richness and precision. For the information richness perspective, HealthQA answer lists critical information for diabetes daily management such as measuring glucose, injecting insulin and exercise. It also mentions the exercise therapy which is not included in the search engine answer. For information precision perspective, although both HealthQA and search engine answers mention oral medications and insulin treatments as diabetes therapies, only HealthQA answer addresses detailed drug class information. Moreover, the search engine answer contains information irrelevant to diabetes medicines and therapies such as diabetes nephropathy. In our manual test, users also prefer the answer given by HealthQA.

Table 6. A sample output of HealthQA

	English	Chinese
Question	Are there any good **medicine** and **therapies** for type II diabetes?	2型糖尿病有什么好**药物**和**治疗方法**?
Health QA Answer	There're no particularly good methods to treat diabetes. Therapies for diabetes include **diet,** physical activity and regular treatments. **For disease management,** all diabetes patients should learn to how to *measure blood glucose,* how to *inject insulin,* how to take *hypoglycemic agen,* as well as the knowledge of *urine glucose, diet* and *exercise.* **Oral medications for diabetes** include insulin secretagogues agent, biguanide, glitazones and AGI. **Insulin treatments** are used for for type I and severe type II diabetes patients. **Exercise therapy** is one method of treatment of diabetes. Proper exercise or physical activity can enhance the peripheral tissue glucose utilization and improve glucose metabolism leading to decreased blood glucose, and thereby achieving therapeutic purposes.	糖尿病目前没什么特别好的办法，主要是**控制饮食**，增加运动量，正规药物治疗。 **一般治疗：**所有糖尿病患者必须进行糖尿病知识普及，使其做到学会*测定血糖*（周围血糖仪法）、*尿糖、注射胰岛素技术、应用饮食、运动、降糖药物的知识和方法。* **口服药物治疗：**促胰岛素分泌剂、双胍类、格列酮类、AGI等。 **胰岛素治疗**适用于1型糖尿病和2型糖尿病的晚期病人。 **运动疗法**是治疗糖尿病的方法之一，通过适当运动或体力劳动，可以增强末梢组织对糖的利用，改善糖代谢使血糖下降，从而提高疗效达到治疗目的。
Search Engine	First, you should know that diabetes is lifetime metabolic disease, which cannot be cured. Even *GBP* can only clinically cure. **Diet therapy**: people with Diabetic Nephropathy (DN) should limit the intake of sodium and protein in the early phase. If necessary, you can transfuse amino acid and plasma. You can take more carbohydrate when on insulin treatment to ensure enough calories intake. If you want to take some fat, better to take from vegetable oil. **Drug therapy**: you can take oral glucose control medications. For the people with renal insufficiency or those who fail to control blood glucose with diet and oral medications, you should consider insulin treatment. Monitor your glucose, and adjust the insulin dosage based on blood glucose level. However, many drugs are toxic, which may cause adverse reactions. So the drugs should be taken properly.	首先您要知道，糖尿病是一种终生性代谢疾病，就目前的医疗水平根本无法彻底治愈糖尿病，就是*胃转流*这种方法也只能达到临床治愈的效果。 **饮食治疗：**目前主张在糖尿病肾病的早期即应限制蛋白质和钠的摄入，争取少而精。必要时可适量输氨基酸和血浆。在胰岛素保证下可适当增加碳水化合物的摄入以保证足够的热量，脂肪宜选用植物油。 **药物治疗：**口服降糖药，对于单纯饮食和口服降糖药控制不好并已有肾功能不全的病人应尽早使用胰岛素。应用胰岛素时需监测血糖及时调整剂量。但是，很多药物中都含有毒成分，会对人的身体带来很大的副作用，要适当的用就行。

5   Conclusion and Future Work

This paper introduced a Chinese QA system for healthcare (HealthQA), which aims at providing people more timely, automatic and valuable QA service than a general search engine. We developed an extended similarity evaluation algorithm to find questions similar to a user query and came up with several significance indicators to evaluate the rank of answers or sentences. Our summarization output is readable and promising.

We will extend this work in the following directions in the future. Our data contains not only the QAs, but also doctors' information. We will use the doctors' information to enhance the evaluation of the reliability of answers. Besides, we will implement topic analysis to get more latent semantic information from the document.

Acknowledgement. This study was supported by the Thousand Talent Program by Tsinghua University, China, National Basic Research Program of China (973 Program) No.2011CB302302 and Tsinghua University Initiative Scientific Research Program. We also appreciate the research assistance provided by Dacheng Zhang from Healthcare Project team in Tsinghua University.

References

1. Athenikos, S.J., Han, H.: Biomedical question answering: A survey. Computer Methods and Programs in Biomedicine 99(1), 1–24 (2010)
2. START, http://start.csail.mit.edu/
3. Kaisser, M.: The QuALiM question-answering demo: Supplementing answers with paragraphs drawn from Wikipedia. In: Proceedings of the 46th Annual Meeting of the Association for Computational Linguistics on Human Language Technologies: Demo Session, pp. 32–35. Association for Computational Linguistics (2008)
4. Radev, D., Fan, W., Qi, H., Wu, H., Grewal, A.: Probabilistic question answering on the web. Journal of the American Society for Information Science and Technology 56(6), 571–583 (2005)
5. Roussinov, D., Fan, W., Robles-Flores, J.: Beyond keywords: Automated question answering on the web. Communications of the ACM 51(9), 60–65 (2008)
6. Lee, M., Cimino, J., Zhu, H.R., et al.: Beyond information retrieval—medical question answering. In: AMIA Annual Symposium Proceedings, vol. 2006, p. 469. American Medical Informatics Association (2006)
7. Cao, Y., Liu, F., Simpson, P., Antieau, L., Bennett, A., Cimino, J., Yu, H.: AskHERMES: An online question answering system for complex clinical questions. Journal of Biomedical Informatics 44(2), 277–288 (2011)
8. Cairns, B.L., Nielsen, R.D., Masanz, J.J., Martin, J.H., Palmer, M.S., Ward, W.H., Savova, G.K.: The MiPACQ clinical question answering system. In: AMIA Annual Symposium Proceedings, vol. 2011, p. 171. American Medical Informatics Association (2011)
9. Ko, J., Si, L., Nyberg, E., Mitamura, T.: Probabilistic models for answer-ranking in multilingual question-answering. ACM Transactions on Information Systems (TOIS) 28(3), 16 (2010)

10. Peng, X., Chen, Y., Huang, Z.: A Chinese Question Answering system using web service on restricted domain. In: 2010 International Conference on Artificial Intelligence and Computational Intelligence (AICI), vol. 1, pp. 350–353. IEEE (2010)
11. Zhang, H., Zhu, L., Xu, S., Li, W.: XML-Based Document Retrieval in Chinese Diseases Question Answering System. In: Park, J.J.(J.H.), Adeli, H., Park, N., Woungang, I., (eds.) Mobile, Ubiquitous, and Intelligent Computing. LNEE, vol. 274, pp. 211–217. Springer, Heidelberg (2014)
12. Meadow, C.T., Boyce, B.R., Kraft, D.H.: Text Information Retrieval Systems, 2nd edn. Academic Press (2000)
13. Lee, M.C.: A novel sentence similarity measure for semantic-based expert systems. Expert Systems with Applications 38(5), 6392–6399 (2011)
14. Caropreso, M.F., Matwin, S., Sebastiani, F.: A learner-independent evaluation of the usefulness of statistical phrases for automated text categorization. In: Text Databases and Document Management: Theory and Practice, pp. 78–102 (2001)
15. Hassan, S., Mihalcea, R.: Semantic Relatedness Using Salient Semantic Analysis. AAAI (2011)
16. Guo, W., Diab, M.: A simple unsupervised latent semantics based approach for sentence similarity. In: Proceedings of the First Joint Conference on Lexical and Computational, pp. 586–590. Association for Computational Linguistics (2012)
17. Li, Y., McLean, D., Bandar, Z.A., et al.: Sentence similarity based on semantic nets and corpus statistics. IEEE Transactions on Knowledge and Data Engineering 18(8), 1138–1150 (2006)
18. Carbonell, J., Goldstein, J.: The use of MMR, diversity-based reranking for reordering documents and producing summaries. In: Proceedings of the 21st Annual International ACM SIGIR Conference on Research and Development in Information Retrieval, pp. 335–336. ACM (1998)
19. Mittal, V., Kantrowitz, M., Goldstein, J., et al.: selecting text spans for document summaries: Heuristics and metrics (1999)
20. Goldstein, J., Mittal, V., Carbonell, J., et al.: Multi-document summarization by sentence extraction. In: Proceedings of the 2000 NAACL-ANLPWorkshop on Automatic Summarization, vol. 4, pp. 40–48. Association for Computational Linguistics (2000)
21. Song, W., Yu, Q., Xu, Z., et al.: Multi-aspect query summarization by composite query. In: Proceedings of the 35th International ACM SIGIR Conference on Research and Development in Information Retrieval, pp. 325–334. ACM (2012)
22. Wang, D., Zhu, S., Li, T., et al.: Multi-document summarization using sentence-based topic models. In: Proceedings of the ACL-IJCNLP 2009 Conference Short Papers, pp. 297–300. Association for Computational Linguistics (2009)
23. Lin, C.Y.: Rouge: A package for automatic evaluation of summaries. In: Text Summarization Branches Out: Proceedings of the ACL 2004 Workshop, pp. 74–81 (2004)
24. Liu, Y., Li, S., Cao, Y., et al.: Understanding and summarizing answers in community-based question answering services. In: Proceedings of the 22nd International Conference on Computational Linguistics, vol. 1, pp. 497–504. Association for Computational Linguistics (2008)

DiabeticLink: An Integrated and Intelligent Cyber-Enabled Health Social Platform for Diabetic Patients

Joshua Chuang[1], Owen Hsiao[2], Pei-Lin Wu[2], Jean Chen[2], Xiao Liu[3],
Haily De La Cruz[3], Shu-Hsing Li[2], and Hsinchun Chen[3]

[1] Caduceus Intelligence Corporation
joshua@caduceusintel.com
[2] National Taiwan University, Taiwan
{owen.w.hsiao,wupeilin.p,trulpa}@gmail.com,
shli@management.ntu.edu.tw
[3] Artificial Intelligence Lab, University of Arizona, United States
{xiaoliu,haily}@email.arizona.edu, hchen@eller.arizona.edu

Abstract. Given the demand of patient-centered care and limited healthcare resources, we believe that the community of diabetic patients is in need of an
integrated cyber-enabled patient empowerment and decision support tool to
promote diabetes prevention and self-management. Most existing tools are scat-
tered and focused on solving a specific problem from a single angle.
DiabeticLink offers an integrated and intelligent web-based platform that enables patient social connectivity and self-management, and offers behavior
change aids using advanced health analytics techniques. DiabeticLink released
a beta version in Taiwan in July 2013. The next versions of the DiabeticLink
system are under active development and will be launched in the U.S., Denmark, and China in 2014. We describe the system functionalities and discuss
the user testing and lessons learned from real-world experience. We also
describe plans for future development.

Keywords: diabetes, patient empowerment, health social media, system
development, user study.

1 Introduction

According to the 2012 annual report of the International Diabetes Federation, 371
million people are living with diabetes all over the world, and more than 471 billion
USD was spent on healthcare for diabetes in 2012 [1]. The prevalence of chronic
diseases such as diabetes has resulted in a severe shortage of healthcare resources,
including health educators, nurses, physicians and hospital beds. Consequently, recent
years have seen increasing interest in patient-centered care and calls to focus on patient empowerment [2]. Diabetes patients are seeking resources for health information
and proper disease management strategies.

The dramatic growth of social media in the past decade has demonstrated its capability to satisfy users' information needs and provide emotional support. The success of

X. Zheng et al. (Eds.): ICSH 2014, LNCS 8549, pp. 63–74, 2014.
© Springer International Publishing Switzerland 2014

health social media sites such as PatientsLikeMe and dailystrength.com shows that there is a new market space for social media patient empowerment tools in the healthcare delivery system to better manage and control patient outcomes. We believe that given the demand of patient-centered care and limited healthcare resources, an integrated cyber-enabled diabetes patient empowerment and decision support tool will help diabetes prevention and management and alleviate some of the pressure on the current healthcare system.

Motivated by these factors, we are developing a patient portal, DiabeticLink, targeting both U.S. and Taiwan audiences, to enable patient social connectivity, and provide personalized healthcare and disease management for diabetes patients with advanced data, text and web mining techniques.

2 Literature Review and Related Systems

There are some existing online social media health websites that offer a subset of the functionalities that DiabeticLink provides. To build the foundation of new features for DiabeticLink, we investigated the existing players in the following areas: diabetes patient portals and online social communities, diabetes tracking and progression visualization, and diabetes risk engines.

2.1 Diabetes Portals and Online Social Communities

Online health social communities provide basic social media functionality such as forums, blogs and member profiles to promote the connection between patients and provide either informational or emotional support through online social networks. Forums allow users to create an online persona (i.e., profile) which affords them anonymity and the ability to connect with other people beyond normal geographic constraints. Some well-established diabetes forums include DiabetesForums.com and tuDiabetes.org.

Satisfying patients' needs for health information is an important goal of existing commercial or non-profit online patient portals. The major players in the diabetes sector are American Diabetes Association (diabetes.org), DiabeticConnect (www.diabeticconnect.com) and DLife (www.dlife.com). They not only include popular social features, but also further provide credible high quality health reference materials such as articles and videos to help newly diagnosed diabetes patients navigate the complex world of active disease management. Other categories of health information on these sites include food intake guides, diabetes recipes, treatment introductions, and local disease support group activities. Most sites rely on manual selection or dedicated writers to create new health information content. None have built mashup applications to aggregate existing high quality diabetes-related content from the web.

2.2   Diabetes Tracking and Visualization

Tracking applications for health and lifestyle factors require a higher level of programming and therefore tend to be independent ventures designed to track diabetic measurements such as blood glucose, Hemoglobin A1c, carbohydrates and physical activity. The current offerings in the market are divided into products that are either: 1) focused on exercise and weight management (e.g., SparkPeople, or MyFitnessPal), or 2) mobile diabetes management systems to track weight, food and activity levels (e.g., Glucose Buddy or OnTrack).

The most popular diabetes tracking mobile apps are Glucose Buddy, Telcare Diabetes Pal, and On Track. These applications differ in user experience, but their functionalities are similar to each other. Glucose Buddy's is the most popular app in terms of total downloads, due to its being one of the oldest diabetic management apps. TactioHealth provides the most comprehensive feature set for diabetics, but it targets a wider audience than just diabetic patients. Its primary benefits are nutrition and weight management. Diabetik is the only app that offers an insulin calculator.

In terms of progression visualization, many tracking applications provide only basic charting. PatientsLikeMe is the only major system that provides a patient with a platform to enter and view his/her own disease data in a more in-depth visualized manner. However, it covers all diseases on one single platform which can be overwhelming and less useful for regular diabetic patients.

2.3   Diabetes Risk Engine

The most important goals of patient empowerment tools are to advance preventative and personalized care, and to foster patients' self-management by raising their awareness of their risks and conditions. To achieve these goals, researchers in both commercial and academic spaces have investigated predictive modeling techniques using longitudinal patient data to predict the risk of a particular patient based on his or her health indicators. The most well-known risk engine is the UKPDS risk engine [4, 5], which predicts heart disease and stroke for type 2 diabetes patients. The current UKPDS risk engine model is built on clinical trial data from 53,000 patients and it predicts the risks for two events only. The adoption and use of electronic health records in clinical practice brings new opportunities to build risk predictive models for a broader range of events for diabetes patients.

2.4   DiabeticLink's Value Proposition

The design of many portals' social features does not promote deeper user interaction through linkage to users' personal health records. Most diabetes tracking apps lack the ability to facilitate users learning from their data. Current diabetes management tools mainly support measuring and tracking. The focus of these apps is on providing a digital logbook, instead of on driving and facilitating improvements in patient health. There is an opportunity to not only provide tracking tools, but to provide tools that will help the user transform their own health-related data into valuable decision-making knowledge.

This knowledge can, in turn, improve the patient's health status by offering data-driven (non-medical) recommendations for small lifestyle changes, such as increasing physical activity or decreasing average carbohydrate levels. Moreover, diabetes apps overall lack features that would directly help or encourage the user to set and monitor long-term goals. Tracking increments in progress towards a goal can prove to be rewarding and motivational for the patient. The Companion App by mySugr [6] is the only app that provides diabetes-specific health recommendations based on the user's data. It primarily targets Type I diabetics. The app sets "challenges" for the user to tackle and monitor. In addition, the tracking process can be more social with peer encouragement and improve user engagement. However, there exists no such application yet.

DiabeticLink enters the diabetes online tools space from a very unique angle in that it offers a more comprehensive suite of tools tailored for diabetic patients than any single existing app to date, including PatientsLikeMe, DiabeticConnect, MyFitnessPal, and GlucoseBuddy. Our system's strength lies in the tools we are creating to aid in patient disease management. Whereas other apps may offer a subset of the features we will release, DiabeticLink will provide an integrated multi-feature social site to patients for total diabetes management as explained above. Our DiabeticLink Tracking module is novel in offering personalized data-based recommendations and progress tracking for goals/challenges. The personalized recommendations with trending and alerting will facilitate better management for disease progression. Gamification (e.g., goals/challenges) will make the self-managing process more sociable and enjoyable. Overall, we envision tracking to be a more social, fun, rewarding and educational experience than it is now.

3 System Functionalities

The current project involves building the DiabeticLink patient portal for both the U.S. and Taiwan audiences. The functionalities of each version are summarized in the following sections.

3.1 DiabeticLink Taiwan Version

To provide our users with a wide range of resources that no current traditional Chinese website for diabetes patients is offering, we organized six main themes with nine different modules in DiabeticLink-Taiwan's website. The six themes are: *1) Health Information; 2) Healthy Diets; 3) Tracking; 4) Knowledge Quick Search; 5) Online Forum; 6) Member Personal Profile.* With these six different themes, our users are able to find accurate and useful information regarding diabetes and healthcare, share their personal experiences, and form an online community. Moreover, they are able to utilize our online diabetes disease management tools to monitor their own biomedical indicators and adjust their lifestyle accordingly. The services DiabeticLink-Taiwan provides are categorized into three main functions in order to serve our users: 1. Education; 2. Social Connections; 3. Online Disease Management Tools. Figure 1 shows the current homepage and an example profile page.

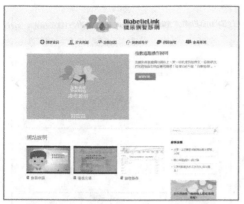 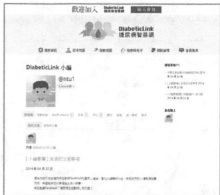

Fig. 1. DiabeticLink-Taiwan *homepage* (left) and *Member Personal Profile* page (right)

Education. DiabeticLink-Taiwan currently provides hundreds of news articles, healthcare and medication related articles, research reports, and healthy diet recipes to our users. The topics of the information range from basic diabetes introductory information, healthy diet, and exercise concepts, to weight control and healthcare knowledge for diabetes patients. Through these articles, our users are able to receive accurate diabetes-related information and form proper healthcare understandings. These contents can be browsed in the *Health Information* and *Health Diets* section.

Moreover, in our *Knowledge Quick Search* section, we also provide resources for the users to search for the answers for some of the frequently asked questions from diabetes patients and their caretakers. For example, our *National Health Insurance Data (NHI) query* module provides answers for the following four types of questions by analyzing the data in the Taiwanese National Health insurance database: 1) the Prevalence of Diabetes in Taiwan, 2) Out-patient Related Questions, 3) Inpatient Related Questions, and 4) Medication Related Questions. Upon using this module, our users are able to get answers for questions such as "What types of insulin does a patient like me take in Taiwan?" and "What is the comorbidity prevalence in Taiwan?"

Social Connections. In our *Online Forum* and *Member Personal Profile* section, we provide forum discussion, personal blog, private messaging, and friending functions to form a friendly environment for our users to create social connections. These social connectivity tools allow users to exchange information, share experiences/concerns, ask and answer questions, and seek mentorship or emotional support without geographic and time zone restrictions, in a synchronous or asynchronous manner.

Online Disease Management Tools. Over the past year, DiabeticLink-Taiwan also adopted two new modules developed in the U.S. and localized the contents to traditional Chinese for our users in Taiwan: *Tracking* and *Drug Safety* modules. The Taiwanese users are now able to utilize the Chinese tracking system to keep track of nine major health related indicators on DiabeticLink-Taiwan. With the new *Tracking* module, shown in Figure 2, diabetes patients can record and monitor their bio-parameters more easily and discover the correlation between their lifestyle and changes of these bio-parameters.

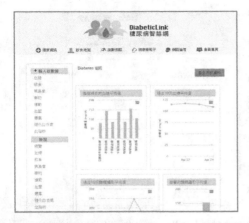
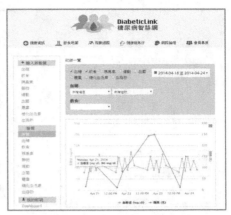

Fig. 2. Tracking module dashboard summary of patient data (left) and bio-parameter correlation summary (right)

Additionally, we also included a total of 139 drugs names that are commonly prescribed to diabetes patients along with their comorbidity from the U.S. Federal Drug Administration (FDA) Adverse Event Reporting System (FAERS) database in the Taiwanese Drug Safety module (Figure 3). The Taiwanese users are able to review the adverse drug effect reports in the FAERS system to have a better understanding of the drugs prescribed to them. For the accuracy of the Chinese translation of these drugs' information, our Taiwanese team consulted with the physicians and educators in National Taiwan University Hospital (NTUH).

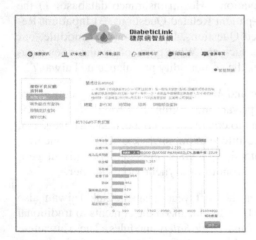
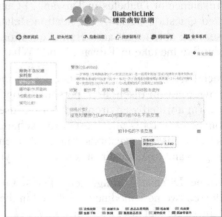

Fig. 3. Adverse Drug Event search (left) and results (right) for Lantus

3.2   DiabeticLink U.S. Version

The functionalities of the U.S. version of DiabeticLink, under development, include a diabetes patient social community, tracking, health information mashup, and a diabetes risk engine.

The **Social Community Platform** is where patients can create a profile and ask questions or make comments on discussion forums, see recent activity and "friend" others to share treatment management questions, experiences, successes, and challenges. Main features include activity feeds, friendships, commenting, user profile, user blog, private messaging, login with Facebook/Twitter, discussion forums, etc.

The **Tracking Module**, shown in Figure 4, allows patients to actively track critical diabetes disease parameters (e.g. Blood Glucose, Blood Pressure, HbA1c, etc.), food/nutrition, physical activity levels, medication and insulin dosage to better manage disease outcomes with visualization to learn their disease progression. The trending dashboard, goal settings, and alerting functions enable users to take proactive actions for managing their conditions, and encourage patient behavior changes.

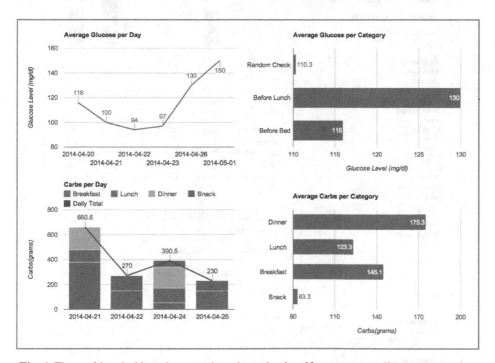

Fig. 4. The tracking dashboard summarizes the patient's self-management disease progression

The **Health Information Mashup Module** focuses on aggregating content from multiple data sources and APIs to create new services for diabetes patients. The major information and services we include in the mashup module can be categorized into general health information, food and nutritional information, treatment information (package insert, FDA's Adverse Event Report and social media adverse event discussions [7]), local support group activities and events, and diabetes-related products and merchandise information. General health information provides an aggregation of diabetes-related news, research, Youtube videos and hot topics from social media platforms such as Facebook and Twitter. Food and nutritional information lists menu items of major chain restaurants and their nutritional facts with geo location information. Treatment information includes the FDA's adverse drug event alert, extracted social media discussions about drug side effects from our analytical tool, and package insert information from the National Library of Medicine. Local disease group activity information aggregates the diabetes local support meetings with events from Meetup.com and Facebook disease support group public pages. Merchandise information provides easy access to diabetes-related products such as books, test strips, and glucometers. The Health Resources mashup delivers up-to-date diabetes-related contents from credible sources based on a user's profile (i.e., location, interests, health conditions, etc.) using advanced data mining, text processing, and machine learning techniques.

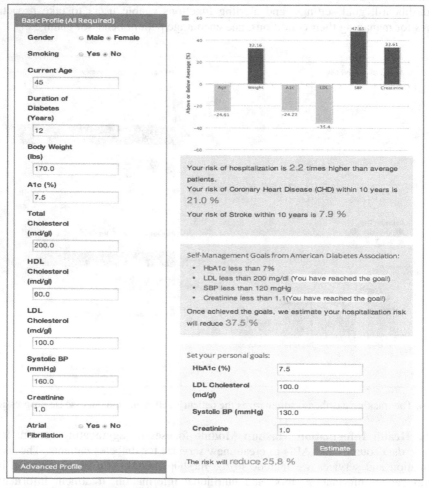

Fig. 5. The Risk Engine prototype, showing the user's current health profile on the left and their risk assessment results and progress toward personal goals on the right

The **Risk Engine** prototypes the research effort developed by the Artificial Intelligence Lab [8] along with a comparison to the UKPDS risk engine to help diabetes patients better understand their risks for hospitalization, stroke, and heart disease so that they may take proper actions to reduce such risks. Figure 5 shows the Risk Engine module, which displays the user's current health profile, progress toward personal goals, and risk assessment results.

4   User Studies and Lessons Learned

The first user test we conducted was for DiabeticLink-Taiwan's beta version release. We collected feedback from both end users and professional personnel regarding their experience of our website and our online tools' features including 1) registration; 2) health information; 3) healthy recipes search; 4) healthy restaurant search; 5) National Health Insurance (NHI) data query; and 6) social forum and member profile. Users not only evaluated the layout, usability, and practicability but also provided their detailed opinions in surveys. The following chart shows the average scores on a five-point rating scale for each section. From the user tests, we found that users valued the relevancy and accuracy of the information on our website. This is shown by the high score of information practicability in each section.

Table 1. Users' Rating for Each Module (Five-point rating scale)

◆ Health Information Resource	
1. Information Practicability	3.42
2. Search function Experience	3.92
3. Layout	3.58
◆ Healthy Recipes Search	
1. Information Practicability	3.83
2. Search function Experience	3.91
3. Layout	3.75
◆ Healthy Restaurant Search	
1. Layout	3.67
◆ NHI Data Query	
1. Information Practicability	3.33
◆ Social Forum	
1. Usability	3.83
2. Layout	3.67
3. Friending Practicability	3.17
4. Topic Subscribing Practicability	4.50

In order to understand users' behavior and reactions toward our *Tracking* module, we also conducted a user test. The current *Tracking* module received 5 out of 6 rating. The high rating shows that the users are satisfied with the features we included in our *Tracking* module. Moreover, the usability of the *Tracking* module, which received 4.9 out of 6 rating, also shows that it had a fairly easy-to-use interface for the users. User suggestions included showing a larger font-size for senior users, providing a mobile app, and integrating with glucometers to reduce user-input errors.

Table 2. Users' Rating for Tracking Module (Six-point rating scale)

◆ Overall Satisfaction	5
◆ Add New Entries	
1. Layout	4.7
2. Usability	4.9
◆ View Entries	
1. Layout	4.85
2. Usability	4.9

5   System Adoption and Usage Statistics

In the nine-month period since July 2013, DiabeticLink-Taiwan attracted more than 33,357 page views with over 6,805 visits, 3,615 unique visitors and 146 registered members. The average visit time was over 4 minutes with 4.9 pages viewed per visit. The Tracking module accounted for 35% of website traffic, followed by static information (17%, including Health Information, Healthy Recipe/Restaurant Search), user test (7%), forum (7%) and others. The fact that our Tracking module attracted 35% of the website traffic shows that the features provided by our Tracking modules show promise for meeting the needs of diabetes patients. From our website analytical tool, we also found that 60% of our users were between the ages of 18 and 34; 33.5% were between 25 and 34; 27.5% were between 18 and 24; and 40% were over 35 years of age. This shows that we are reaching primarily a younger population. As a result, we are also utilizing current social media such as a Facebook fan page to promote our website and to reach a greater number of potential users.

6   Future Development Plans

In July 2013, DiabeticLink-Taiwan released its beta version and became the first diabetes social media platform in Taiwan. With production experience and lessons learned from DiabeticLink-Taiwan, DiabeticLink-U.S. is under active development for a new version to be publicly released in August 2014. Meanwhile, DiabeticLink-Denmark, a collaborative effort with the Patient@home program, has been planned for late 2014. Patient@home is Denmark's largest welfare-technological research and innovation initiative with a focus on new technologies and services within the Danish public health sector [9].

After the first year of website operations, we now have a better understanding of the needs of the diabetes patients and other user groups. In the future, DiabeticLink-Taiwan will continue collecting and providing users with relevant and accurate information from credible sources. Furthermore, in order to develop new online disease management tools for patients that are more in line with clinical practices, we have started collecting feedback from medical personnel including physicians, registered nurses, and educational personnel within the endocrinology departments of various hospitals in Taiwan. Due to the day-to-day contact with actual diabetic patients, these personnel have the potential to provide new insights and valuable feedback to the DiabeticLink website and the ongoing development of our online tools.

Mobile app development and integration with the portal is essential, i.e., mobile access and data synchronization. The Tracking module will be integrated with mobile devices, allowing patients to use their phone or tablet or the web application to manage disease and lifestyle factors. Automatic data capture (e.g., Bluetooth) is also being considered.

Being the information and data hub, the interoperability of the system with third party medical or fitness tracking devices is also essential. The "Quantified-Self" movement [10] is happening rapidly in the fitness and exercise space as the technology is maturing. Not only are big companies such as Nike, Sony, and Samsung showing interest and investing in this space, but many startup companies, such as FitBit, Jawbone, and Moves (acquired by Facebook), are also pushing the movement forward. We believe, with this trend, that it is beneficial for diabetes patients to adopt new technologies and help live a healthier lifestyle. Many vendors have also released APIs for data integration. Withings Body Metrics Services API [11], for instance, allows access to health data measured by their products, including weight, blood pressure, heart rate, etc. We plan to integrate with such vendors' APIs for streamlining user data capture and being part of the bigger ecosystem.

We will also explore possible automatic approaches for content categorization, which will classify the latest diabetes information into categories such as news, research, diet, etc. We plan to develop more customized subscription functions for users to follow specific topics that they are interested in and allow users to comment, like and interact with others on our site. Other future developments may include enhanced visualization, analytics tools, integrated dashboard, and workflow improvement with care providers.

Acknowledgement. This work is supported in part by the University of Arizona Artificial Intelligence Lab (DTRA award #HDTRA1-09-1-0058), the Caduceus Intelligence Corporation, and the National Taiwan University. We wish to acknowledge our collaborators in both the U.S. and Taiwan.

References

1. International Diabetes Federation Annual Report,
   http://www.idf.org/sites/default/files/IDF_Annual_Report_
   2012-EN-web.pdf

2. Greaves, F., Ramirez-Cano, D., Millett, C., Darzi, A., Donaldson, L.: Harnessing the cloud of patient experience: using social media to detect poor quality healthcare. BMJ Quality & Safety 22(3), 251–255 (2013)
3. Chen, H., Compton, S., Hsiao, O.: DiabeticLink: A Health Big Data System for Patient Empowerment and Personalized Healthcare. In: Zeng, D., Yang, C.C., Tseng, V.S., Xing, C., Chen, H., Wang, F.-Y., Zheng, X. (eds.) ICSH 2013. LNCS, vol. 8040, pp. 71–83. Springer, Heidelberg (2013)
4. Stevens, R.J., Kothari, V., Adler, A.I., Stratton, I.M.: The UKPDS Risk Engine: a model for the risk of coronary heart disease in Type II diabetes (UKPDS 56). Clinical Science 101(6), 671–679 (2001)
5. Kothari, V., Stevens, R.J., Adler, A.I., Stratton, I.M., Manley, S.E., Neil, H.A., Holman, R.R.: UKPDS 60: risk of stroke in type 2 diabetes estimated by the UK Prospective Diabetes Study risk engine. Stroke; a Journal of Cerebral Circulation 33(7), 1776–1781 (2002)
6. Companion App by mySugr, https://mysugr.com/companion/
7. Liu, X., Chen, H.: AZDrugMiner: an information extraction system for mining patient-reported adverse drug events in online patient forums. In: Zeng, D., Yang, C.C., Tseng, V.S., Xing, C., Chen, H., Wang, F.-Y., Zheng, X. (eds.) ICSH 2013. LNCS, vol. 8040, pp. 134–150. Springer, Heidelberg (2013)
8. Lin, Y.-K., Chen, H., Brown, R.A., Li, S.-H., Yang, H.-J.: Time-to-Event Predictive Modeling for Chronic Conditions using Electronic Health Records. IEEE Intelligent Systems (forthcoming, 2014)
9. Patient@home, http://www.en.patientathome.dk/
10. Technology Quarterly. The quantified self, counting every moment, technology and health: measuring your everyday activities can help improve your quality of life, according to aficionados of "self-tracking". The Economist (2012), http://www.economist.com/node/21548493
11. Withings API, http://www.withings.com/api

Collaborative Friendship Networks in Online Healthcare Communities: An Exponential Random Graph Model Analysis

Xiaolong Song[1], Shan Jiang[2], Xiangbin Yan[1], and Hsinchun Chen[2]

[1] School of Management, Harbin Institute of Technology, Harbin, China
xlsong45@gmail.com, xbyan@hit.edu.cn
[2] Department of Management Information Systems, University of Arizona,
Tucson, United States
jiangs@email.arizona.edu, hchen@eller.arizona.edu

Abstract. Health 2.0 provides patients an unprecedented way to connect with each other online. However, less attention has been paid to how patient collaborative friendships form in online healthcare communities. This study examines the relationship between collaborative friendship formation and patients' characteristics. Results from Exponential Random Graph Model (ERGM) analysis indicate that gender homophily doesn't appear in CFNs, while health homophily such as treatments homophily and health-status homophily increases the likelihood of collaborative friendship formation. This study provides insights for improving website design to help foster close relationship among patients and deepen levels of engagement.

Keywords: Health 2.0, Patient networks, Collaborative friendship, ERGMs.

1 Introduction

The core concept of Health 2.0 is using Web 2.0 technologies to support better healthcare [42]. It provides patients an unprecedented opportunity to connect with each other, and enables them to gain social support and improve health collectively in long-term. Compared to other forms of social relationships in online context, virtual friendship in health social media is created based on a common goal that patients collaborate in expectation of positive changes in health condition. Therefore in this paper, we use the term "collaborative friendship" to describe this type of virtual friendship in online health social media.

Users in health social media generally differ in individual characteristics and health-related interests, which influence the way in which patients develop social ties. However, it is unclear how various patients form collaborative friendship online. Prior studies generally attribute the formation of social ties to homophily that the similarities of individual attributes lead people to build close relationship [1, 2, 3]. In a health social media context where improving health condition is a central concern, patients are motivated to find others who have experienced or are suffering from similar health problems. The challenge is that the similarity may stem from various aspects of individual health, such as health condition and treatment experience. Nevertheless, what type of and to what extent homophily leads to collaborative friendship are still unknown.

X. Zheng et al. (Eds.): ICSH 2014, LNCS 8549, pp. 75–87, 2014.
© Springer International Publishing Switzerland 2014

In this study, we utilize a theory-grounded statistical modeling approach—Exponential Random Graph Model (ERGM) to investigate what aspect of individual characteristics affect the formation of collaborative friendship network (CFN) in online healthcare communities. The study provides insights for improving Health 2.0 websites design to help foster close relationship among patients and deepen levels of engagement.

2 Literature Review

Our work draws from two streams of literature. We first summarize recent studies on patient networks in online healthcare communities. Then we review the how the core analytical methodology, ERGMs, has been used in prior social network research.

2.1 Patient Networks in Online Healthcare Communities

Online healthcare communities are emerging as a collection of individuals who have common healthcare interests. Patient network analysis is suggested by Chen et al. [4] as one of the most promising areas for health information technology research. Table 1 summarizes previous online patient networks studies based on the types of relationships between users, the directions of the research, the factors that affect the formation of social ties, and analytical approaches used in the studies.

Table 1. Summary of Selected Patient Networks in Online Health Communities Studies

Literature	Types of Relationships	Research Direction	Types of Affecting Factors on Tie formation	Analytical Approaches
Chang (2009)	Communication	Network characteristics	N/A	Network structural analysis
Ma et al. (2010)	Friendship	Network characteristics	N/A	Network structural analysis
Durant et al. (2010)	Communication	Network characteristics	N/A	Network structural analysis
Centola (2010)	Friendship	Network influence	N/A	Social experiment
Centola (2011)	Friendship	Network influence	N/A	Social experiment
Yan et al. (2011)	Subscription	Tie formation	Actor-attributes, Structural dependency	Logistic regression
Stewart et al. (2012)	Communication	Network characteristics	N/A	Network structural analysis
Durant et al. (2012)	Communication	Tie formation	Actor-attributes	Network structural analysis
Chomutare et al. (2013)	Communication	Network characteristics	N/A	Network structural analysis
Chuang et al. (2013)	Communication	Network characteristics	N/A	Blockmodel

As Table 1 shown, network influence, network structure characteristics, and tie formation are the three most adopted major research directions. The network influence study focuses on how online social networks influence changes in health behavior [8, 9]. Most of the studies listed in Table 1 can be classified as network characteristics research, which generally describes the structural characteristics of the patient network and the positions of individuals [6], [10], [11], [12], [13]. The tie formation studies mainly examine what determinants influence the formation of patients' connection. For instance, Durant et al. has found that patients preferred to communicate with other patients with the same gender [14]. While prior study focuses on the formation of patient communication relationship [14] and patient subscription relationship [15], little research has been done to understand how collaborative friendship ties form in the online healthcare setting.

Recent studies have identified a variety of factors that potentially influence the formation process of patient network ties. These factors can be categorized into structural dependencies and actor-attributes. Structural dependencies are endogenous network structure-based effects. By contrast, actor-attributes refer to individual characteristics of patients, independent of their connections. The actor-attributes of a patient can be generally divided into two aspects: health-related attributes and demographic attributes. Both types of attributes could influence the formation of patient relationships in online healthcare communities [14, 15].

Several types of analytical approaches have been used in prior patient networks literature. Social experiment provides a controlled approach to test how behaviors are influenced by specific factors. Blockmodels can be constructed to perform position analysis. But both of the methods above have limitations in dealing with multiple attributes of network nodes (i.e. patients). To examine the structural characteristics of patient networks, most prior studies tend to use network structural analysis. However, it is hard to determine the causality between non-structural factors (e.g. individual health condition) and tie formation. The logistic regression model with random effect is recently used to examine multiple attributes simultaneously with relations and introduce a random effect to control for interdependency among the dyad observations latently [15].

2.2 Exponential Random Graph Models

In this study, to examine how patient CFN forms we adopt a theory-grounded probabilistic social network modeling approach – Exponential random graph models [16, 17] for the following reasons. First, unlike most general linear models with the independence assumption, ERGMs assume the interdependencies of network ties. ERGMs can also induce features and dependencies with multi-dimensions simultaneously and explicitly capture the interdependency of relational data by measured covariates [18]. These strengths enable the ERGMs to deal with network data where nodes (i.e. patients in the context of CFN) have multiple attributes and formation of ties is interrelated.

The general mathematical form of exponential random graph models is as follow:

$$Pr(\mathrm{Y}{=}\mathrm{y}) = \frac{1}{\kappa}\exp\left\{ \sum_{A}\eta_A g_A(\mathrm{y}) \right\},$$ (1)

where the summation in the model is over all configurations. η_A is the parameter corresponding to configuration A. $g_A(y)$ indicates the network statistic. κ is a normalizing quantity to ensure proper probability distribution. A configuration is a subset of possible network ties [17].

Aiming at finding the network model which can best describe the observed network, the ERGMs generate random networks based on network statistics measured from an observed network and then compare them. The more similar the structure of the observed network and the random networks is, the better the ERGM estimations are. The estimated parameters in the final fitted model will indicate whether some of the configurations (i.e. network patterns) are statistically frequently observed: a positive (negative) significant parameter would suggest that the corresponding network pattern is more likely (unlikely) to occur.

As mentioned above, with the exceptions of Durant et al. (2012) [14] on communication networks and Yan et al. (2011)'s work [15] on subscription networks, no research has examined the formation mechanism of patient networks, especially patient CFN. Further, a network-based approach that has the capability to deal with multiple attributes of nodes and the interdependency of network ties is needed.

To fill these gaps, we propose the following research questions: How do patients build collaborative friendships in online healthcare communities? What types of homophily influence the formation of collaborative friendships in online healthcare communities?

3 Theory and Research Hypotheses

To answer these questions, several hypotheses are developed based on the Theory of Homophily.

Theory of Homophily

According to the theory of homophily, social ties are more likely to occur between individuals with common features or similar attributes [1]. Empirical evidences indicate that there are a variety of homophily, in terms of race [3], gender [2], and so on. Prior explanation of homophily phenomena highlights the positive relationship between the perceived similarity and the preference for social contact [23, 24]. Shared characteristics could lead to identification, which increases the tendency of making strong connections [25].

Regarding friendship networks, existing evidences reveal that the similarity based on demographic attributes like gender are well-established factors affecting friendship formation [1], [26]. The study of health social networks requires health-relevant traits like health status [22], [27]. Therefore, there may be two types of homophily which correspond to the two aspects of a patient's actor-attributes: demographic homophily and health homophily. To identify what types of shared health attributes could lead to health homophily, we should understand the motivation of patients' online friendship seeking behaviors. Prior studies have indicated that the most popular topics drawing online patients' attention are treatments and health condition [28, 29]. Thus we examine the potential roles of health-homophily based on treatments and health condition on the formation of CFNs.

Demographic Homophily
As mentioned above, the gender is critical for the development of offline social ties [1]. Men and women tend to differ in the cognitive process and healthcare behaviors. For example, women often pay more attention to weight-control and are more likely to be on a diet than men [19].

However, increasing evidence shows that the communication in online social media breaks the gender boundary. For instance, a study on patient subscription network has found that there was no gender homophily in an online mental health community [15]. Thus we expect that gender homophily has little influence on patient CFN formation in online healthcare communities[1].

Hypothesis 1: The effect of gender-homophily on collaborative friendship formation is insignificant.

Treatment Homophily
Seeking detailed information about treatments is one of the main purposes of patients using health social media [20]. Individuals typically desire the information about the risk, benefits, and uncertainty related to treatments [21]. Patients with shared treatments tend to face similar problems and have the same types of information needs. Also, newly diagnosed patients often take plenty of time to accumulate experiences so that they can effectively self-manage their treatments. The treatment experience of others can be seen as an important reference. Therefore, patients are more likely to develop social ties with others sharing the same treatments.

Hypothesis 2.1: Patients with the same treatments tend to establish collaborative friendships.

Besides current treatments, patients also desire information about other potential treatment options [30]. First, patients may pay attention to some potential activities for supplementing their current activities [31]. Also, the evolution of the illness or the appearance of complications may lead to the treatment changes. Meanwhile, the bigger the difference in the number of treatments between two patients, the more likely they differ in health condition. For the safety and efficacy, patients are more likely to learn experience from others with a similar number of treatments. Recent evidence shows that the similar number of treatments has a positive influence on the formation of patient subscription relationships [15]. Therefore, we propose the following hypothesis:

Hypothesis 2.2: Sharing similar number of treatments increases the probability for patients to establish collaborative friendships.

Health Condition Homophily
Health condition generally includes disease severity and disease duration [32]. On one hand, according to social comparisons theory [33], individuals are likely to compare themselves to other patients to evaluate their health condition and to learn from others who are better off than them [34, 35]. Therefore, similarity in health status should be

---

[1] Here we focus on general chronic illness with little gender-specific differences in treatments.

positively related to the likelihood of forming collaborative friendship. On the other hand, benefits from being friends with patients who are in poor condition may be limited. Patients tend to perform activities that they believe would improve their health [36], patients with good health status are thus more attractive for social contacts. Collaborative friendship is a relationship of mutual preference, and thus a collaborative friendship with a poor-conditioned patient might not be proactively sought. Combining the aforementioned two arguments, we propose the following hypothesis.

Hypothesis 3.1: Patients in good health status are likely to build collaborative friendships.

As the other dimension of health condition, disease duration is the time passed since the point of diagnosis. For chronic illness, disease duration is often related to complications. For instance, it is hard to see complications in Type 1 diabetes patients with disease duration of less than 5 years [37]. Similarity in disease duration enables patients with the same illness more comparable [38, 39]. By comparing with each other, patients could better understand how well they are doing. Therefore we hypothesize that:

Hypothesis 3.2: Patients with similar disease duration are likely to form collaborative friendships.

4   Research Design

We propose a framework for the ERGM-based analysis in this study, which is illustrated in Figure 1.

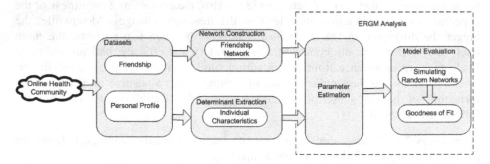

Fig. 1. Research Framework

In order to test our hypothesis, data was collected from TuDiabetes (http://www.tudiabetes.org/), a worldwide online diabetes community launched in 2007. The online platform integrates a range of online healthcare services which not only allows its members to create online profiles and discuss in forums, but also develop "friend" relationship, which provides a perfect context for studying the formation of CFNs.

In this study, we focus on patients with type 1 (which includes LADA) diabetes which is the largest group of diabetic patients among others as our research test-bed. Two sets of information were collected: (a) We obtained all the profile information of these users who joined the community by July 5, 2013; (b) We also extracted all the friendship data of these users during the time. We dropped the records of users who haven't contributed anything to forums discussion. We also removed individual records with missing value. Finally, the process resulted in a dataset of 2118 users and 4134 friendship ties.

Determinants were extracted from the profile information of our data to capture individual characteristics. In the diabetic context, we identified a patient as having good health status if her HbA1C% is greater than or equal to 7%. The value is suggested by the American Diabetes Association as the target for most non-pregnant adults with diabetes[2]. We used the difference of the year of diagnosis to measure the similarity of disease duration. Considering high changes in year level due to scaling effect, we applied the log transformation.

For applying ERGMs, configurations were constructed to represent various hypothesized dependencies. Table 2 summarizes the research hypotheses, parameters used, and the corresponding configurations. Generally, a significant positive parameter will suggest that the corresponding configuration is more likely to occur in the network than by chance, which in turn supports the corresponding hypothesis. The parameter [treatment/duration]-difference measures the absolute difference between two actor attributes for continuous attributes. Therefore for hypotheses 2.2 and 3.2, if the corresponding parameters are negative and significant, it will suggest that two nodes with less absolute difference in attributes tend to form ties, which in turn supports the corresponding hypotheses. As suggested by Robins (2011) [17], we also included the network statistic – edges as a control variable which can be seen as an intercept term that accounts for the number of the edges in the network.

We estimated the parameters associated with hypotheses with Markov Chain Monte Carlo maximum likelihood estimation (MCMCMLE) methods, as suggested by prior studies [17, 18]. With the algorithm, the network statistics will converge when the parameters best represents the observed network.

In order to validate how well the ERGMs fit the observed network, we conduct a goodness-of-fit test. We generated 100,000,000 simulated networks.1000 samples were picked up to compare with the observed network in a series of network statistics. Low difference in the statistics of the observed network and generated samples would indicate a fit of the estimated model.

---

[2] http://www.diabetes.org/living-with-diabetes/treatment-and-care/blood-glucose-control/checking-your-blood-glucose.html/

Table 2. Research Hypothesis, Parameter and Configuration

Hypothesis	Parameter	Configuration
Hypothesis 1: The effect of same-gender on collaborative friendship formation is insignificant.	[gender]-interaction	 male(female) male(female)
Hypothesis 2.1: Patients with same treatments tend to establish collaborative friendships.	[treatment]-matching	 treatment A treatment A
Hypothesis 2.2: Sharing similar number of treatments increases the probability for patients to establish collaborative friendships.	[number of treatment]-difference	 x treatments y treatments (x≥y)
Hypothesis 3.1: Patients in good health status are likely to build collaborative friendships.	[good health status]-interaction	 good health status good health status
Hypothesis 3.2: Patients with similar disease duration are likely to form collaborative friendships.	[diagnosis duration]-difference	 x years after diagnosis y years after dianosis (x≥y)

5   Results and Discussion

5.1   Results Analysis

Table 3 reports the results of ERGM estimates and hypotheses testing. Following prior studies, a parameter was considered significant if the value of the estimate was at least twice the standard error [43, 44].

The parameter estimate for demographic homophily was not significant, indicating that gender has little influence on collaborative friendship formation, which supports H1. This finding provides new evidence to support the previous finding that gender homophily does not always appear in social media [40].

H2.1 was supported, providing evidence that having the same current treatments is an important motivating factor for making friends. Treatment experience information from online peers with same treatments can reduce the uncertainty. Well-informed patients tend to have a positive effect on treatment outcomes [21]. The parameter estimate for H2.2 was significant but negative, indicating that two patients with great absolute difference in the number of treatments tended to build collaborative friendship. This was contrary to our hypothesis, and thus H2.2 was not supported. This observation implies that patients may build collaborative friendships with others who have more experiences in the disease in order to seek help and learn from their experiences.

Table 3. Results of ERGM Estimates

Type	Hypothesis	Estimate	Std dev	t-statistics	Result
Demographic homophily	H1	0.086700	0.17196	0.04368	Supported
Treatment experience homophily	H2.1	0.255650*	0.05300	-0.05804	Supported
	H2.2	0.209109*	0.01900	-0.00381	NOT supported
Health condition homophily	H3.1	0.506711*	0.15458	-0.03431	Supported
	H3.2	-2.094521	2.68512	-0.04568	NOT supported

Notes:
   t-statistics = (observation - sample mean)/standard error. Low t-statistics indicate that the parameter is converged in the MCMCMLE process.

H3.1 was supported, indicating that patients in good health status in online healthcare communities are more likely to develop collaborative friendship with each other. Relations in patient friendship networks are mutually agreed-upon. Both sides expect to benefit from their friendship. Therefore, patients in relatively poor health condition are less attractive for patients with good health status. The finding is consistent with De La Haye et al. (2011)'s study [22] that health status similarity can affect friendship selection in real world.

Similar disease duration exhibits an insignificant effect, suggesting that similar disease duration doesn't increase the probability of forming social ties. Therefore, H3.2 was not supported. The lack of support for the hypothesis could be that the effect of similar disease duration on collaborative friendship formation could be mixed. People with short disease duration also need know about preventing complications and make friends with those who have longer illness experience.

In sum, our study explains how CFNs form and why patients turn to CFNs. First, patients determine whom they should connect to without thinking about gender, which could facility the flow of health-related knowledge within a wider range in CFNs. Second, treatments homophily and health-status homophily have been found in online healthcare communities. Patients require a tailored online environment which can positively influence their healthcare behaviors. In order to acquire effective and consistent peer support, patients value others who have similar health status and build collaborative friendships with them. Current treatment and health status can predict the formation of friendship.

5.2   Goodness of Fit Tests

Table 4 shows the goodness of fit testing results for a variety of network statistics. If the absolute value of a t-ratio is less than 0.1, the model can be seen as a good fit for the data [45]. In our case, with the exception of [number of treatment]-difference and [good health condition]-interaction, most of parameters were less than 0.1. The results indicate that though the model was capable to reproduce most of the properties in the observed network well, there was space for improving the model fitness by including more factors that may affect the formation of CFN.

Table 4. Results of Goodness-of-fit Test

Parameter	Observed value	Mean	Std dev	t-Ratio
Edge	3183	3182.971	40.949	0.001
[gender]-interaction	43	42.876	6.899	0.018
[treatment]-matching	580	581.523	21.783	-0.070
[number of treatment]-difference	4233	4206.319	74.253	0.359
[good health status]-interaction	61	60.223	6.898	0.113
[diagnosis duration]-difference	23.993	23.978	0.493	0.031

Notes:
t-Ratio = (observation - sample mean)/standard error

6   Conclusion

Understanding how patient characteristics affect CFNs formation is vital to the growth and success of health social media. Health-homophily such as treatment homophily and health-status homophily can increase the likelihood of collaborative friendship formation. Taking account of these factors can help health social media designers promote users' socialization and increase the level of participation.

Our study contributes to both streams of literature of social media and healthcare. We examine how patients form CFNs in online healthcare communities, which fills the gaps in a growing literature of online patient networks. We use a theory-grounded statistical modeling approach – EGRMs, to demonstrate the capability of dealing with patient network data. We find the formation of collaborative friendship is driven by health-homophily, which provides new evidence to homophily theory. The results of this study also have important practical implications for website providers and health behavior intervention strategies. Our study provides insights into enhancing friend-seeking service to facilitate patients' socialization. For instance, online healthcare communities can provide users with tools to search others by treatment information.

The limitation of this study is that we only examined the patient friendship formation in a diabetes setting. Further work will extend to broader contexts such as general chronic diseases.

References

1. McPherson, M., Smith-Lovin, L., Cook, J.M.: Birds of a feather: Homophily in social networks. Annual Review of Sociology, 415–444 (2001)
2. Ibarra, H.: Homophily and differential returns: Sex differences in network structure and access in an advertising firm. Administrative Science Quarterly 37, 422–447 (1992)
3. Mollica, K.A., Gray, B., Trevino, L.K.: Racial homophily and its persistence in newcomers' social networks. Organization Science 14, 123–136 (2003)
4. Chen, H., Chiang, R.H.L., Storey, V.C.: Business intelligence and analytics: From big data to big impact. MIS Quarterly 36, 1165–1188 (2012)
5. Monge, P.R., Contractor, N.S.: Theories of communication networks. Oxford University Press, New York (2003)
6. Stewart, S.A., Abidi, S.S.R.: Applying Social Network Analysis to Understand the Knowledge Sharing Behaviour of Practitioners in a Clinical Online Discussion Forum. Journal of medical Internet research 14, e170 (2012)
7. Granovetter, M.S.: The strength of weak ties. American Journal of Sociology, 1360–1380 (1973)
8. Centola, D.: The spread of behavior in an online social network experiment. Science 329, 1194–1197 (2010)
9. Centola, D.: An experimental study of homophily in the adoption of health behavior. Science 334, 1269–1272 (2011)
10. Chang, H.J.: Online supportive interactions: using a network approach to examine communication patterns within a psychosis social support group in Taiwan. Journal of the American Society for Information Science and Technology 60, 1504–1517 (2009)
11. Durant, K.T., McCray, A.T., Safran, C.: Social network analysis of an online melanoma discussion group. In: AMIA Summits on Translational Science Proceedings (2010)
12. Chomutare, T., Årsand, E., Hartvigsen, G.: Characterizing development patterns of healthcare social networks. Network Modeling Analysis in Health Informatics and Bioinformatics, 1–11 (2013)
13. Chuang, K.Y., Yang, C.C.: How do e-patients connect online? a study of social support roles in health social networking. In: Greenberg, A.M., Kennedy, W.G., Bos, N.D. (eds.) SBP 2013. LNCS, vol. 7812, pp. 193–200. Springer, Heidelberg (2013)
14. Durant, K.T., McCray, A.T., Safran, C.: Identifying gender-Preferred communication styles within online cancer communities: A retrospective, longitudinal Analysis. PloS One 7, e49169 (2012)
15. Yan, L., Tan, Y., Peng, J.: Network dynamics: How can we find patients likeus? Available at SSRN (2011),
http://papers.ssrn.com/sol3/papers.cfm?abstract_id=1820748
16. Wasserman, S., Pattison, P.: Logit models and logistic regressions for social networks: I. An introduction to Markov graphs and p. Psychometrika 61, 401–425 (1996)
17. Robins, G.: Exponential random graph models for social networks. In: Handbook of Social Network Analysis. Sage (2011)
18. Handcock, M.S., Hunter, D.R., Butts, C.T., Goodreau, S.M., Morris, M.: Statnet: Software tools for the representation, visualization, analysis and simulation of network data. Journal of Statistical Software 24, 1548 (2008)
19. Wardle, J., Haase, A.M., Steptoe, A., Nillapun, M., Jonwutiwes, K., Bellisie, F.: Gender differences in food choice: the contribution of health beliefs and dieting. Annals of Behavioral Medicine 27, 107–116 (2004)

20. Sugawara, Y., Narimatsu, H., Hozawa, A., Shao, L., Otani, K., Fukao, A.: Cancer patients on Twitter: a novel patient community on social media. BMC Research Notes 5, 699 (2012)

21. Charnock, D., Shepperd, S., Needham, G., Gann, R.: DISCERN: an instrument for judging the quality of written consumer health information on treatment choices. Journal of Epidemiology and Community Health 53, 105–111 (1999)

22. De La Haye, K., Robins, G., Mohr, P., Wilson, C.: Homophily and contagion as explanations for weight similarities among adolescent friends. Journal of Adolescent Health 49, 421–427 (2011)

23. Byrne, D.: Attitudes and attraction. Advances in Experimental Social Psychology 4, 35–89 (1969)

24. Huston, T.L., Levinger, G.: Interpersonal attraction and relationships. Annual Review of Psychology 29, 115–156 (1978)

25. Mehra, A., Kilduff, M., Brass, D.J.: At the margins: A distinctiveness approach to the social identity and social networks of underrepresented groups. Academy of Management Journal 41, 441–452 (1998)

26. Shrum, W., Cheek Jr., N.H., MacD, S.: Friendship in school: Gender and racial homophily. Sociology of Education, 227–239 (1988)

27. Smith, K.P., Christakis, N.A.: Social networks and health. Annual Review of Sociology 34, 405–429 (2008)

28. Diaz, J.A., Griffith, R.A., Ng, J.J., Reinert, S.E., Friedmann, P.D., Moulton, A.W.: Patients' use of the Internet for medical information. Journal of General Internal Medicine 17, 180–185 (2002)

29. Shuyler, K.S., Knight, K.M.: What are patients seeking when they turn to the Internet? Qualitative content analysis of questions asked by visitors to an orthopaedics Web site. Journal of Medical Internet Research 5 (2003)

30. Pereira, J.L., Koski, S., Hanson, J., Bruera, E.D., Mackey, J.R.: Internet usage among women with breast cancer: an exploratory study. Clinical Breast Cancer 1, 148–153 (2000)

31. Knowler, W.C., Barrett-Connor, E., Fowler, S.E., Hamman, R.F., Lachin, J.M., Walker, E.A., Nathan, D.M.: Reduction in the incidence of type II diabetes with lifestyle intervention or metformin. New England Journal of Medicine 346, 393–403 (2002)

32. Guo, S.E., Huang, C.Y., Hsu, H.T.: Information needs among patients with chronic obstructive pulmonary disease at their first hospital admission: priorities and correlates. Journal of Clinical Nursing (2013)

33. Festinger, L.: A theory of social comparison processes. Human Relations 7, 117–140 (1954)

34. Helgeson, V.S., Taylor, S.E.: Social comparisons and adjustment among cardiac patients1. Journal of Applied Social Psychology 23, 1171–1195 (1993)

35. Wood, J.V., VanderZee, K.: Social comparisons among cancer patients: under what conditions are comparisons upward and downward? In: Health, Coping, and Well-being, pp. 299–328 (1997)

36. Harris, D.M., Guten, S.: Health-protective behavior: An exploratory study. Journal of Health and Social Behavior, 17–29 (1979)

37. King, R.A., Rotter, J.I., Motulsky, A.G.: The genetic basis of common diseases. Oxford University Press (2002)

38. Gordon, P., West, J., Jones, H., Gibson, T.: A 10 year prospective followup of patients with rheumatoid arthritis 1986-96. The Journal of Rheumatology 28, 2409–2415 (2001)

39. Van Gaalen, F.A., Toes, R.E., Ditzel, H.J., Schaller, M., Breedveld, F.C., Verweij, C.L., Huizinga, T.W.: Association of autoantibodies to glucose-6-phosphate isomerase with extraarticular complications in rheumatoid arthritis. Arthritis & Rheumatism 50, 395–399 (2004)
40. Thelwall, M.: Homophily in myspace. Journal of the American Society for Information Science and Technology 60, 219–231 (2008)
41. Ma, X., Chen, G., Xiao, J.: Analysis of an online health social network. Paper presented at the Proceedings of the 1st ACM International Health Informatics Symposium (2010)
42. Van De Belt, T.H., Engelen, L.J., Berben, S.A., Schoonhoven, L.: Definition of Health 2.0 and Medicine 2.0: a systematic review. Journal of Medical Internet Research 12, e18 (2010)
43. Pahor, M., Škerlavaj, M., Dimovski, V.: Evidence for the network perspective on organizational learning. Journal of the American Society for Information Science and Technology 59, 1985–1994 (2008)
44. Su, C., Contractor, N.: A multidimensional network approach to studying team members' information seeking from human and digital knowledge sources in consulting firms. Journal of the American Society for Information Science and Technology 62, 1257–1275 (2011)
45. Snijders, T.A.B.: Markov chain Monte Carlo estimation of exponential random graph models. Journal of Social Structure 3, 1–40 (2002)

The Impact of Alcohol Intake
on Human Beings Health in China

Wenbin Wang, Kaiye Gao[*], and Qing Wei

Dongling School of Economics and Management,
University of Science and Technology Beijing, Beijing, 100083, China
gaokaiye1992@qq.com

Abstract. Drinking is one of the main causes of disease burden. In this paper, we tried to find the effect of alcohol intake on health state using the China Health and Nutrition Survey data in a model of regression. We initially used the self assessed health, which was widely used in related studies, in the database as the health variable but obtained controversial result. After that, to test the result we compared the drinking status between participants who are longevous and who are not and found the initial result is unreasonable. We then used the life span as our health variable which produced sensible result as expected. Linear regression and ordinal logistic regression were used to quantify the effect of alcohol intake on health. The results for our sample suggest two conclusions: 1) drinkers are overconfident in their health statuses; and 2) alcohol intake does shorten the life span on average.

Keywords: Alcohol intake, Life span, Health, Regression.

1   Introduction

Alcohol intake is the world's third largest risk factor for disease burden. The harmful use of alcohol results in 2.5 million deaths each year. 320000 young people between the age of 15 and 29 die from alcohol-related causes, resulting in 9% of all deaths in that age group, [1]. There are many health complications associated with alcohol abuse, such as illnesses of the liver and pancreas, malnutrition, and fetal abnormalities. Patients taking heavy alcohol have more than eight times risk on progression to cirrhosis than that taking a normal level of alcohol of the same age at infection, [2]. Youth with recent alcohol use tend to experience a poorer level of health-related quality of life, [3]. In a 12-year prospective study, Newcomb and Bentler found that adolescent alcohol and drug use had deteriorating effects on later adult mental health, such as an increase in depression, anxiety, and suicide ideation, [4].

Alcohol drinkers, including those with heavy drinking, reported better self-assessed health(SAH) related quality of life than nondrinkers in Spain [5]. They found out such conclusion, but did not investigate that the drinkers are indeed healthier than

---

[*] Corresponding author.

X. Zheng et al. (Eds.): ICSH 2014, LNCS 8549, pp. 88–96, 2014.

non-drinkers. In this paper we found that the trend of life span are different from the trend of SAH among participants in drinking status.

The main objective of this paper is, however, try to identify and quantify the relationship between drinking and health using a database in China. To observe the trend of the relationship, we classified levels of drinking by alcohol intake. There are many reported papers about how and how much the alcohol intake can damage our health, [2,3,4]. While there are fewer papers about how drinkers assess about their health. There is a SAH variable in the database so initially we tried to use the SAH to study the impact of drinking on human health. However, because of the bias in SAH described earlier, the use of SAH as the health variable did not support our intended hypothesis that drinking impairs the health. Whereupon we divided participants into two groups which are the longevous and the short-lived to see the difference of alcohol intake between them. Then we used the life span which is age at death as our health variable and the result is supportive. In Section 2, we will give a introduction of the study sample we used. Then we proceed to the variable selection and methods in Section 3. The result is presented in Section 4 and Section 5 concludes the paper.

2   Study Sample

Details of the China Health and Nutrition Survey (CHNS) are described in [6]. Briefly, this Survey was started in 1989 by the Carolina Population Center at the University of North Carolina at Chapel Hill and the National Institute of Nutrition and Food Safety at the Chinese Center for Disease Control and Prevention. The aim of the CHNS is see how the social and economic transformation of Chinese society is affecting the health and nutritional status of its population, [7]. The survey took a 3-day period using a multistage, random cluster process to draw a sample of about 4400 households with a total of 26,000 individuals in nine provinces, which is the representative of the whole country in geography, stages of economic development, levels of living condition and health status both physically and psychologically. There are nine waves in the cohort, which are 1989, 1991, 1993, 1997, 2000, 2004, 2006, 2009 and 2011.

The data is longitudinal in nature. One participant in one wave generates one row of record in the data table. We used all participants to describe a roughly trend of the influence of alcohol intake in health. The dead were extracted from the longitudinal data. And we used the latest record of the dead to find the influence of drinking on life span.

3   Variables and Methods

3.1   Drinking Status

Average alcohol intake was obtained by asking individuals about their alcohol consumption statuses in a typical week during the last year. The total weekly amount of pure alcohol consumption was not directly taking from the data. We converted the consumption of beer, grape wine and liquor to the pure alcohol consumption. Finally, The average daily intake of pure alcohol(ADI) was calculated by dividing the total weekly amount of pure alcohol by 7 days, see equation (1). We classified the levels of drinking as non-drinking, light drinking and heavy drinking by ADI. Drinkers whose average daily intake of pure alcohol are more than 50ml were defined as heavy drinkers. The rest of drinkers were defined as light drinkers.

$$I = \frac{I_b \times C_b + I_g \times C_g + I_l \times C_l}{7},$$ (1)

Notation

I ADI
I_b Weekly intake of beer
I_g Weekly intake of grape wine
I_l Weekly intake of liquor
C_b Beer-alcohol concentration
C_g Grape wine-alcohol concentration
C_l Liquor-alcohol concentration

3.2   Health Variable

Our initial thought about the health variable is the SAH. The SAH, [8], refers to a survey indicator commonly used in health research in which participants are invited to assess the aspect of their own health condition. The SAH was typically structured using a Likert Scale. It has become an increasingly common measure used in surveys among the ageing and patients with chronic diseases. The question of the SAH in the questionnaire of CHNS is "Right now, how would you describe your health condition when compared to those in your age?". The answers are "1. excellent; 2. good; 3. fair; 4. poor; 9 unknown". Literally, the SAH had eliminated the influence of age. It reflects a person belief about his or her health condition which is often used in the health related study, [5].

In the database there are some recorded deaths, so the life span can be another health variable to be used with the assumption that if a person lived longer, he or she will be regarded healthier than those died earlier. It is an objective measure of a person's health.

3.3   Methods

In the present study, we first used the descriptive statistics to analyze the rough trend and the direction of the effects of the alcohol intake on SAH and life span. Then we used the ordinal logistic regression to calculate the effect of alcohol intake on the SAH and then the longevity since the SAH and longevity is categorical variable. Next, we used the linear regression to calculate the exact effect of alcohol intake on life span. Linear regression is perhaps the simplest but effective means to quantify the relationship between a dependent variable such as life span and independent variable such as alcohol intake with the hypothesis that alcohol intake can shorten one's life.

4   Results

4.1   Data Review

A total of 94,490 records of 27,703 participants were included in the present analysis. Of the initial sample of 27,703 participants, 24,313 reported drinking status and the SAH. Among these participants, 1,265 have a death record. The summary of the data is shown in Table 1.

Table 1. Characteristics of participants with different drinking status

No.	Variables	0.Non-drinkers	1. Light drinkers	2. Heavy drinkers
All participants				
	Age			
1	16-19	3714	334	47
2	20-29	8312	1866	606
3	30-39	9561	2579	1365
4	40-49	9754	2819	1793
5	50-59	8293	2227	1412
6	60-69	5942	1341	715
7	70-79	3337	606	284
8	80-	961	134	38
Deaths among participants				
	Lifespan			
1	16-19	11	1	0
2	20-29	43	9	3
3	30-39	52	18	8
4	40-49	79	30	17
5	50-59	156	40	23
6	60-69	261	58	36
7	70-79	353	59	26
8	80-	276	32	13
	SAH			
1	excellent	18	6	7
2	good	162	42	25
3	fair	231	59	25
4	poor	207	20	10
Longevity(>76y)				
0	No(<76y)	511	117	82
1	Yes(>76y)	501	106	35

4.2   SAH

Since SAH is categorical variable so we used ordinal logistic regression to quantify such relationship between alcohol intake and SAH but obtained controversial result. As the SAH of their health are different at each survey, we used the SAH in his or her latest survey.

As we can see in Figure 1 and Table 1, the proportion of drinkers among participants with excellent and good SAH status is larger than those with fair and poor SAH. So we can see that the drinkers have a relatively better SAH than the non-drinkers. The ordinal logistic regression of SAH and ADI also confirmed this conclusion, see Table 2.

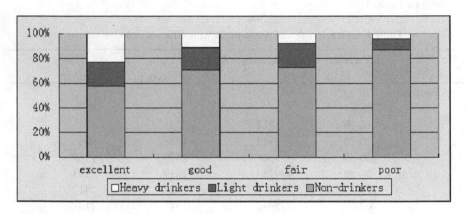

Fig. 1. Proportion of drinking at different ranks of SAH

Table 2. Coefficients of ordinal logistic regression in SAH

Coefficients	Estimate	Std. Error	z value	Pr(>|z|)
β (ADI)	-0.005741	0.001658	-3.463	0.000535 ***
α_1 (SAH 1|2)	-3.33241	0.18684	-17.84	
α_2 (SAH 2|3)	-0.83837	0.07956	-10.54	
α_3 (SAH 3|4)	0.82019	0.07940	10.33	

Asterisks *** indicate statistical significance at the 1% level.

According to the cumulative probability formula of ordinal logistic regression:

$$P(y \le j \mid x = i) = \frac{1}{1 + \exp(\beta \times i - \alpha_j)},$$ (2)

We can derive the probability   of each level of SAH, see equations (3) and (4).

$$P(y = j \mid x = i) = P(y \le j \mid x = i) - P(y \le j-1 \mid x = i),$$ (3)

$$
\begin{cases}
P(y=1\,|\,x=i)=\dfrac{1}{1+\exp(\beta\times x-\alpha_1)},\ y=1 \\[2ex]
P(y=j\,|\,x=i)=\dfrac{1}{1+\exp(\beta\times x-\alpha_j)}-\dfrac{1}{1+\exp(\beta\times x-\alpha_{j-1})},\ y=2,3 \\[2ex]
P(y=4\,|\,x=i)=1-\dfrac{1}{1+\exp(\beta\times x-\alpha_3)},\ y=4
\end{cases}
$$

$$(4)$$

The probability of each rank of SAH at different levels of drinking can be calculated by equations (3) and (4) and the results are shown in Table 3. Non-drinkers (ADI=0) are more likely to report poor or fair health. While drinkers (ADI>0) are more likely to report excellent or good health and heavy drinkers (ADI>50) have more chances to do that than light drinkers (0<ADI<=50).

Table 3. The logical probability of each rank of SAH at each level of drinking

ADI/SAH	1. Excellent	2. Good	<=2	3. Fair	4. Poor
0	0.03447592	0.26740227	0.3018782	0.39239848	0.30572333
15	0.03746025	0.28286990	0.3203301	0.39191331	0.28775654
30	0.04069203	0.29866967	0.3393617	0.39020396	0.27043435
45	0.04418982	0.31473703	0.3589268	0.38728980	0.25378335
60	0.04797323	0.33099967	0.3789729	0.38320371	0.23782338
75	0.05206293	0.34737803	0.399441	0.37799130	0.22256774
90	0.05648058	0.36378579	0.4202664	0.37171002	0.20802361

4.3 Longevity

In this part, since we can observe whether participants are longevous or not so we want to find the difference in drinking status between participants who are longevous and those who are not. Longevity is defined as a person living exceed 76 years old (The life expectancy of Chinese). The participants who are not longevous come from those with records death at age before 76. The participants who are longevous come from the participants who are lived over 76 years old, included the dead and those still alive.

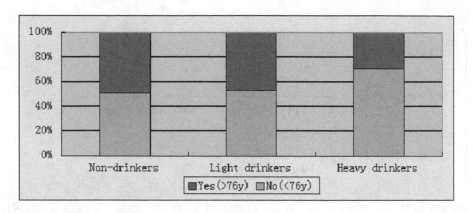

Fig. 2. Proportion of participants who are longevous or not

Figure 2 show that participants who are longevous are less likely drinking than participants who are not.

Just as what we did in the SAH part, ordinal logistic regression was used in longevity by ADI. Since theories are the same as SAH part so they were omitted here. The probability of being a longevous man among participants are shown in Table 4.

Table 4. The probability of whether being a longevous man or not

No.	Longevous	0.Non-drinkers	1.Light drinkers	2.Heavy drinkers
0	No(<76y)	0.4215	0.4992	0.5769
1	Yes(>76y)	0.5785	0.5008	0.4215

As is shown in Table 4, drinkers have less chances to live longer than 76 years than non-drinkers. And heavy drinkers have least chances to live longer than 76 years than light drinkers and non-drinkers. It also mirrors that drinkers have poor health in general.

4.4   Life Span

To examine the association between alcohol intake and life span, we selected participants who had already died in the tracking studies.

As we can see in Figure 3 and Table 1, among those with a recorded death, there were more drinkers in the 30-69 life spans and then substantially decreased for those lived longer 70 years. It seemed that non-drinkers will live longer than drinkers. Because some younger people died accidentally, we excluded those whose life spans were less than 50 years in the subsequent analysis.

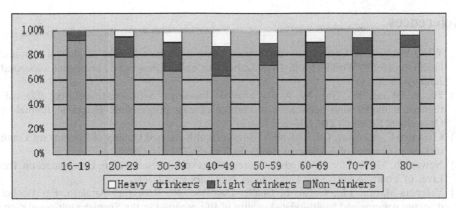

Fig. 3. Proportion of drinking at each cohort of life span

Table 5. Results of linear regression

Coefficients	Estimate	Std. Error	t value	Pr(>|t|)
Intercept	75.8089	0.310894	233.067	< 2e-16 ***
ADI	-0.036474	0.008141	-4.481	8.08e-06 ***

Asterisks *** indicate statistical significance at the 1% level.

We can see in the result of the linear regression shown in Table 5 that each one more milliliter of ADI will decrease life span about 0.036474 years(13 days).

5   Conclusion

The results indicate that each one milliliter increasing of ADI will decrease the life span about 13 days but increase the probability of having a good or excellent SAH. Non-drinkers have less chances to live longer than 76 years than drinkers. Thus it can be concluded that drinkers are overconfident in their health status.

We should let drinkers know that alcohol intake can injure their health undoubted. In some cases, they are falling to recognise that they are not healthy. The damage of alcohol intake is a process from quantitative change to qualitative change. The key to stay healthy is to have regular medical checkup and keep the healthy lifestyle, since prevention is better than cure.

Acknowledgement. The research report here was partially supported by the NSFC under grant number 71231001, China Postdoctoral Science Foundation funded project under Grant 2013M530531, the Fundamental Research Funds for the Central Universities of China under grant numbers FRF-MP-13-009A and FRF-TP-13-026A, and by the MOE PhD supervisor fund, 20120006110025.

We are grateful to all the volunteers who participated in CHNS. There would be no data reported herein without them.

References

[1] WHO Framework Convention on Tobacco Control: Is harmful use of alcohol a public health problem? World Health Organization, http://www.who.int/en/ (accessed January 28, 2014)

[2] Fu, B., Wang, W., Shi, X.: A risk analysis based on a two-stage delayed diagnosis regression model with application to chronic disease progression. European Journal of Operational Research 218, 847–855 (2012)

[3] Chenand, C.-Y., Storr, C.L.: Alcohol Use and Health-Related Quality of Life among Youth in Taiwan. Journal of Adolescent Health 39, 752.e9–752.e16 (2006)

[4] Newcomb, M., Bentler, P.M. (eds.): Consequences of Adolescent Drug Use: Impact on The Lives of Young Adults. Sage Publications, Newbury Park (1998)

[5] Valencia-Martín, J.L., Galán, I., Guallar-Castillón, P., Rodríguez-Artalejo, F.: Alcohol drinking patterns and health-related quality of life reported in the Spanishadult population. Preventive Medicine 57, 703–707 (2013)

[6] Popkin, B.M., Du, S., Zhai, F., Zhang, B.: The China Health and Nutrition Survey: monitoring and understanding socioeconomic and health change in China 1989-2011. Int. J. Epidemiol. 39, 1435–1440 (2010)

[7] China Health and Nutrition Survey.: China Health and Nutrition Survey, http://www.cpc.unc.edu/projects/china/ (accessed January 28, 2014)

[8] Fayers, P.: Assessing Quality Of Life In Clinical Trials: Methods And Practice. Oxford University Press, Oxford (2005)

Social Support and User Engagement in Online Health Communities

Xi Wang, Kang Zhao, and Nick Street

The University of Iowa
{xi-wang-1,kang-zhao,nick-street}@uiowa.edu

Abstract. Online health communities (OHCs) have become a major source of social support for people with health problems. Members of OHCs interact online with those who face similar problems and are involved in different types of social supports, such as informational support, emotional support and companionship. Using a case study of an OHC among breast cancer survivors, we first use machine learning techniques to reveal the types of social support embedded in each post from an OHC. Then we generate each user's contribution profile by aggregating the user's involvement in various types of social support and reveal that users play different roles in the OHC. By comparing online activities for users with different roles and conducting survival analysis on users' time span of online activities, we illustrate that users' levels of engagement in an OHC are related to various types of social support in different ways.

Keywords: Social Support, Online Health Communities, User Engagement, Survival Analysis, Text Mining.

1 Introduction

Nowadays more and more people use the Internet to satisfy their health-related needs. According to a study by the Pew Research Centre, 80% of adult Internet users in the U.S. use the Internet for health-related purposes. Among them, 34% read health-related experiences or comments from others [1]. Compared with traditional health-related websites that only allow users to retrieve information, online health communities (OHCs) increased members' ability to interact with peers facing similar health problems and as a result better meet their immediate needs for social support. It is estimated that 5% of all Internet users participated in an OHC [2].

While people use OHCs for a wide range of needs, obtaining psychosocial support is one of the key benefits of engagement in OHCs [3,4]. Research has found that such support can help patients adjust to the stress of living with and fighting against their diseases [5,6,7] and is a consistent indicator of survival [8]. An OHC also serves as an outlet for users' emotional needs and improve their offline life [9]. Thus active engagement in an OHC has been found to be therapeutic to users [10] and it is important to keep users engaged in the community.

X. Zheng et al. (Eds.): ICSH 2014, LNCS 8549, pp. 97–110, 2014.

Literature on social support suggests that OHCs mainly feature three types of social support: informational support, emotional support, and companionship (a.k.a., network support) [11,12]. *Informational support* is the transmission of information, suggestion or guidance to the community users [13]. The content of such a post in an OHC is usually related to advice, referrals, education and personal experience with the disease or health problem. Example topics include side effects of a drug, ways to deal with a symptom, experience with a physician, or medical insurance problems. *Emotional support*, as its name suggests, contains the expression of understanding, encouragement, empathy affection, affirming, validation, sympathy, caring and concern, etc. Such support can help one reduce the levels of stress or anxiety. Companionship or network support consists of chatting, humour, teasing, as well as discussions of offline activities and daily life that are not necessarily related to one's health problems. Examples include sharing jokes, birthday wishes, holiday plans, or online scrabble games. Companionship helps to strengthen group members' social network and sense of communities.

Previous studies of OHCs have examined social support among OHC members. For instance, the qualitative study by Zhang et al. [14] found that users exchange *informational support* more frequently than other types of social support in an OHC for smoking cession. Nambisan [15] indicated *informational support* and social support existing in OHCs, but the information seeking effectiveness affects patient's perceived empathy. By contrast, Ahmed et al. [16] suggested that peer-to-peer information support is the key aspect for a Facebook group related to concussion.

Then is a user's involvement in and exposure to different types of social support related to her/his engagement in an OHC? Few studies have answered this question systematically by examining users' seeking, receiving, and provision of various types of social support. A previous study showed that users who received more emotional support tended to stay longer, while receiving more informational support does not keep a user engaged [17]. However, the study did not consider companionship or users' roles and behaviors in seeking and providing support.

In this research, we addressed three research questions regarding social support and user engagement in OHCs: (1) Can we use machine learning techniques to detect the seeking and provision of three major types of social support embedded in interactions among users; (2) Are there any patterns of users' involvement in different types of social support activities? Or in other words, do users play different roles when it comes to seeking and providing social support? And (3) Are the seeking, providing, and exposure to different types of social support related to users' engagement in an OHC? The outcome of this research has implications for building and sustaining an active OHC through better thread/post recommendations and community management.

2 Detecting Social Supports from Texts

2.1 Dataset and the Taxonomy of Social Support

In this research, we used Breastcancer.org as a case study. It is a very popular peer-to-peer OHC among breast cancer survivors and their caregivers. With more than

140,000 registered users, the website provides various ways for its members to communicate, including discussion forums, private messaging, friend subscriptions, listserv, etc. We designed a web crawler to collect data from its online forum, which has 73 discussion boards. Our dataset consists of all the public posts and user profile information from October 2002 to August 2013. There are more than 2.8 million posts, including 107,549 initial posts. These posts were contributed by 49,552 users.

Table 1. Example posts for types of social support

Social Support Category	Examples
Companionship (COM)	*Kelly Have a wonderful time in Florida, enjoy the sun and fun. Heather* *I'm loving her new CD. Didn't recognize any of the songs at first, but there are a few now that I find myself singing the rest of the day.* *This game has the poster making a new 2 word phrase starting with the second word of the last post Example: Post : Hand out Next poster: Out cast Next poster: Cast Iron Next poster: Iron Age Now let's begin the game~ Age Old*
Seeking Informational Support (SIS)	*Where do you buy digestive enzymes and what are they called?*
Seeking Emotional Support (SES)	*I feel like everyone else's lives are going forward, they have plans, hopes, aspirations because they feel. I am one of those not yet out of the woods. I was also someone who could never get cancer. I was a good person, exercised, ate well. Good people don't get sick. I have taken the step of antidepressants, they mitigate the damage, but do not block the pain or sadness I feel.*
Providing Informational Support (PIS)	*I had surgery Aug05 for bc recurrance. B4 surgery I had 33 IMRT rads, prior to that had 4A/C & 4 Taxol. I had bc in 2000 & had 37 rads in same general area. Now, my surgery won't heal. Wound doc says there is adema or something on my sternum (shown on recent MRI). My wound has been draining since it broke open in Sept.*
Providing Emotional Support (PES)	*Hope you feel better soon, we are here! Prayers Hugs come from Massachusetts APPLE♥.*
Providing Informational Support (PIS) & Providing Emotional Support (PES)	*I am also the daughter of a 35 yrs BC survivor. Mom is just now going through some more Cancer - alas - they found it in her lung, but it is totally unlikely to be a follow-up of her old BC. I am 45, and was 43 at DX time, my mom was diagnosed at 38... and I am a BRCA2 carrier. Tina, one day at a time. Maybe you'll get good news - it is so hard to wait!!! It is also important to remember that - whatever it is, it is highly treatable, and that YOU WILL SURVIVE too!!! and life goes on after. It will take some time, but it goes on... see my picture? even the hair is back!!! Hugs to all. I am happy you all found your way here, it is a great site for exchanging information, learning and finding support.*

As we mentioned earlier, informational support, emotional support, and companionship are the three major types of social supports in OHCs. Thus for each post, we need to determine whether it was seeking informational support (SIS), providing informational support (PIS), seeking emotional support (SES), providing emotional support (PES), or simply about companionship (COM). Note that we did not differentiate seeking and provision of companionship, because the nature of companionship is about participation and sharing. By getting involved in activities or discussions about companionship, one is seeking and providing support at the same time. It is also possible that a post could belong to more than one of the categories above. Table 1 lists example posts for each category and a post that belongs to two categories.

2.2   Annotations and Features

As it is almost impossible to label all 2.8 million posts manually, we used classification algorithms to decide what kind(s) of social support each post contains. To train the classification algorithm, we leveraged human annotated data. We randomly selected 1,333 (54 initial posts and 1,279 comments) out of our dataset. After basic training on the aforementioned five categories of social supports (SIS, PIS, SES, PES, COM), five human annotators were asked to read each post and decide whether the post is related to one or more categories of social supports.

To control the quality of human annotations, we also added to the pool 10 posts that have been annotated by domain experts. For each post, we only accepted results from annotators whose performance on the 10 quality-control posts is among top 3. Results from the other two annotators were discarded. Then a majority vote was used to determine whether a post is related to a category of social support. Table 2 shows the results of the annotation process.

Table 2. The number of posts in each category of social support in the annotated dataset

Social Support Category	Number
Companionship (COM)	435
Seeking Informational Support (SIS)	96
Seeking Emotional Support (SES)	22
Providing Informational Support (PIS)	411
Providing Emotional Support (PES)	249

Users in OHCs may have different writing styles or linguistic preferences to express themselves. To capture these characteristics, we examined each post and extracted various types of features for the classifier: basic features, lexical features, sentiment features, and topic features. Table 3 summarizes these features. Many of the features were picked specifically for classification in this context. For example, we included whether a post is an initial post as a feature because many users seek support by starting a thread. Inside each post, the existences of URLs and emoticons are often related to informational and emotional supports respectively. Similar to the approach used by [17], we also checked the usage of phrases in the format of <you/he/she + MODAL verb > to express possibilities, such as "you should", "she could". We considered "he" and "she" in addition to "you", because some posts were created by family members of cancer survivors. To identify the difference between "seeking" and "providing" support, we included words related to seeking behaviour, such as "question", "wonder" and "anybody". We also hoped that words related to daily life topics and geographical locations can effectively detect companionship. Meanwhile, we used OpinionFinder [18] to find the overall sentiment, as well as subjectivity and objectivity of each post. Besides these handpicked or dictionary-based lexicons, we also wanted to capture whether the usage of other words and phrases can contribute to the classification. Using unigrams and bigrams is too fine-grained and leads to a feature set with very high dimension. Thus we adopted an approach similar to [17] and applied topic-modelling technique Latent Dirichlet Allocation (LDA, with k=20) [19] to the content of all posts and generated 20 topics. For each post, LDA gave a topic probability distribution, indicating the probability of this post corresponding to each topic. Such a distribution for each post was then included in the feature set.

Table 3. Summary of features for the classifier

Group	Features
Basic Features	Whether the post is an initial post in a thread
	Whether the post is a self reply
	Length of the post
Lexical Features	Whether the post contains URLs (Y or N)
	Whether the post contains emoticon(s)
	Number of numeric numbers
	Number of Pronouns (e.g., they, we, I)
	Whether the post contains the negation word(s) (e.g., not, never, no)
	Whether the post contains name(s) of city, state, country (U.S.A, Canada, etc.)
	Whether the post contains phrases related to possibility (you must, you might, she had better, etc.)
	Whether the post contains names of drugs related to breast cancer (From http://www.cancer.gov/cancertopics/druginfo/breastcancer)
	Whether the post contains breast cancer terminology (From http://www.breastcancer.org/dictionary)
	Whether the post contains verb related to advice (Need, require, recommend, etc.)
	Whether the post contains emotional words (Love, sorry, hope, worry, etc.)
	Whether the post contains words related to seeking behaviours (Anybody, question, wonder, etc.)
	Whether the post contains words related to daily life topics (Vacation, joke, run, walk, etc.)
Sentiment Features	Frequency of words with positive and negative sentiment
	Objectivity and subjectivity scores
Topic Features	Topic distributions derived from LDA

2.3   Evaluation of the Classifier

Because there are five categories of social supports and a post may be related to more than one category, we built a classifier for each category. For the classification of each category of social support, we applied various classification algorithms on annotated posts and picked the best performing algorithm (using 10-fold cross-validation). Because posts seeking emotional support accounted for only a small proportion among annotated posts (22 out of 1,333), we oversampled posts seeking emotional support when building the SES classifier. Table 4 compares the performance of different algorithms for the five categories of social support. AdaBoost was chosen to classify COM, PES[1], PIS and SIS, while logistic regression was the best choice for SES. Overall, our classifiers achieved decent performance with accuracy rate over 0.8 in all five classification tasks.

Table 4. Performance of classification algorithms for five categories of social supports

Social support	Results	Naïve Bayes	Logistic Regression	SVM (Poly Kernel)	Random Forest	Decision Tree	AdaBoost
COM	Accuracy	0.696	0.787	0.783	0.771	0.767	**0.804**
	ROC Area	0.839	0.817	0.768	0.848	0.75	**0.852**
PES	Accuracy	0.713	0.830	0.840	0.830	0.81	**0.817**
	ROC Area	0.823	0.787	0.681	0.825	0.687	**0.817**
PIS	Accuracy	0.753	0.813	0.823	0.767	0.779	**0.801**
	ROC Area	0.824	0.83	0.783	0.837	0.717	**0.859**
SES	Accuracy	0.893	**0.901**	0.970	0.967	0.963	0.963
	ROC Area	0.749	**0.867**	0.656	0.851	0.671	0.668
SIS	Accuracy	0.851	0.880	0.943	0.931	0.937	**0.914**
	ROC Area	0.893	0.803	0.745	0.86	0.766	**0.869**

After applying the best-performing five classifiers on the remaining of the 2.8 million posts, each post received 5 labels, each of which indicates whether the post belong to one of the five social support categories. The total numbers of posts in each category are listed in Table 5.

Intuitively, there are more posts to provide support than to seek support. This is what most would expect from a popular OHC with a large and active user base. About 37% of the posts provided informational support, making it the largest group among the five. In other words, providing informational support is the most popular activity in the OHC. Companionship posts constitute the second largest group, which suggests that members of the OHC did form a strong sense of community and discussed many issues other than cancer.   In addition, 197,956 posts were predicted to provide informational and emotional support at the same time, representing the largest group with more than one category of social support.

---

[1] Although the results of accuracy and ROC area of random forest are slightly better than AdaBoost for the PES classifier, the random forest classifier has much worse recall and f-measure. Thus we decided to choose AdaBoost.

Table 5. Total numbers of posts in each category of social supports

Social support category	Number of posts
Companionship (COM)	932,538
Seeking Informational Support (SIS)	284,027
Seeking Emotional Support (SES)	227,188
Providing Informational Support (PIS)	1,034,682
Providing Emotional Support (PES)	497,096

3   User Profiling and Engagement

After estimating the nature of social support in each post, we can then build a profile for each user by aggregating her/his posts by their social support categories. We represented each user's social support involvement with a 1×5 a vector. Each element in the vector is the percentage of the user's posts in a social support category. For example, user Mary has published 10 posts, with 3 companionship posts, 4 posts providing emotional support, 2 posts providing informational support, 1 post seeking emotional support, and no posts seeking informational support. Then she will have a vector of <0.3, 0.4, 0.2, 0.1, 0>.

With social support distribution vectors of 47,581 users, we applied the classic K-means clustering algorithm to divide users into k groups, so that the users with similar social support distributions would belong to the same cluster. To find the best grouping of users, we tested various K values (from 2 to 20) and clustering results with Davies-Bouldin Index (DBI) [20]. DBI is defined as Equation 1, where $D_{intra}(C_i)$ is the average distance from all the other users in cluster C_i to the centroid of C_i, and $D_{inter}(C_i, C_j)$ is the distance between centroids of C_i and C_j. Euclidean distance was used for this study. Generally speaking, DBI prefers smaller groups, for the value of intra-cluster distance is lower in the smaller group, and penalizes short inter-cluster distances. Therefore, the solution with the lowest DBI provides relative balance of small clusters and long distances between every pair of clusters.

$$DBI = \frac{1}{k}\sum_{i=1}^{k} max_{j:i\neq j}\left\{\frac{D_{intra}(C_i)+D_{intra}(C_j)}{D_{inter}(C_i,C_j)}\right\} \qquad (1)$$

We summarized the DBIs for different K values in Table 6. K=7 yielded the lowest DBI value and hence the best clustering results. Centroids for each of the 7 clusters are shown in Table 7.

From Table 7, we can see that, intentionally or not, OHC users do have different patterns in social support involvement and thus play different roles in the community. Some users' posts focused on one major category of social support. For example, users in cluster 0 published an average of 96.55% of their social support posts to provide informational support. They obviously act as *information providers* in the community. Similarly, cluster 1 is for *community builders* with 64.92% of supports in companionship, and cluster 4 consists of *emotional support providers*. The two smallest clusters are for seekers: cluster 3 for *information seekers* and cluster 6 for *emotional support seekers*. Meanwhile, users in cluster 2, the largest cluster of the seven, are *all-around contributors* with relatively balanced profiles in each social support category. Cluster 5 represents a group of *information enthusiasts*, who focus mainly on informational support, both seeking and providing.

Next we investigated how users in different groups engaged in the OHC. Engagement levels were measured by two metrics: productivity (i.e., a user's total number of posts) and time span of activities (i.e., the number of days between a user's first and last post). Fig 1(a) compares the distributions of productivity for users in the 7 clusters. The curves suggest that community builders in cluster 1, albeit a small group of users, and all-around contributors in cluster 2 are the most productive members. By contrast, those who mainly seek support (informational or emotional) in clusters 3 and 6 published fewer posts than others. Fig 1(b) points to similar conclusions: those in clusters 1 and 2 stayed with the community for the longest time, while support seekers in clusters 3 and 6 have relatively short time span of activities. Overall, those who are more actively involved in companionship tend to get engaged in the community, while those who only seek support are more likely to "churn". Also, emotional support providers in cluster 4 are more engaged that information providers in cluster 0.

Table 6. The DBIs for the K-means clustering with various K values

K	DBI	K	DBI
2	1.485806117	12	0.932705779
3	1.183743056	13	0.914857805
4	1.147831469	14	1.148624229
5	1.002816698	15	0.94766141
6	0.962159462	16	0.915504995
7	0.89111499	17	0.895295641
8	0.977535018	18	0.907029696
9	0.960697173	19	0.935044276
10	0.940555275	20	1.001204328
11	0.904557568		

Table 7. Centroids of user clusters

Social Support	All users	Cluster 0	Cluster 1	Cluster 2	Cluster 3	Cluster 4	Cluster 5	Cluster 6
COM	0.1126	0.0042	0.6492	0.1271	0.0154	0.0504	0.0408	0.0404
PES	0.1178	0.0074	0.0833	0.1511	0.0053	0.612	0.0315	0.0351
PIS	0.4422	0.9655	0.1277	0.4762	0.0152	0.2394	0.4369	0.0325
SES	0.0743	0.0067	0.0349	0.1245	0.0107	0.0481	0.0494	0.5868
SIS	0.2531	0.0162	0.1049	0.1211	0.9534	0.0501	0.4414	0.3052
# of users	47581	6647	3923	15336	3502	3994	13225	954
% of users		14%	8%	32%	7%	8%	28%	2%

To better clarify the differences among the clusters, we use two-sample Kolmogo-rov-Smirnov test (K-S test) to compute the statistical gaps between every two clusters in both productivity and time span of activities. Two-sample K-S test, which is used to compare whether two one-dimensional probability distributions are different, is defined as

$$D_{n,n'} = \sup|F_{1,n}(x) - F_{2,n'}(x)| \qquad (2)$$

where $F_{1,n}(x)$ and $F_{2,n'}(x)$ are the empirical distributions of a metric for two groups. The closer the result is to 0, the more likely the two samples are drawn from the same distribution. In Table 8, the upper triangular matrix (shaded area) shows the K-S statistics for comparing productivities between every pair of user clusters, and the lower triangular matrix shows the K-S statistics for time spans. For both metrics, the difference between clusters 2 and 3 is the greatest, which is consistent with what we observed in the Fig 1. In addition, p-values for all K-S tests are less than to 0.001, suggesting statistically significant differences among all clusters' distributions of both engagement metrics.

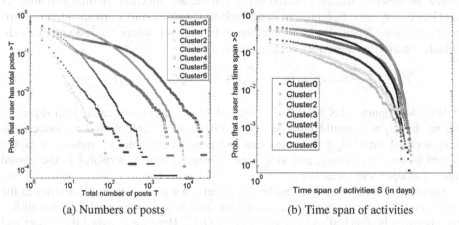

(a) Numbers of posts   (b) Time span of activities

Fig. 1. Complementary cumulative distributions of engagement metrics for the users in different clusters

Table 8. K-S statistics on engagement metrics for each pair of user clusters. The shaded area is for the comparison on number of the posts. The unshaded area is for time span of activities. All values are significant at p=0.001.

	Cluster 0	C 1	C 2	C 3	C 4	C 5	C 6
Cluster 0	-	0.329	0.660	0.056	0.235	0.358	0.062
C 1	0.278	-	0.348	0.321	0.148	0.178	0.301
C 2	0.602	0.348	-	0.673	0.465	0.409	0.653
C 3	0.080	0.320	0.665	-	0.219	0.317	0.071
C 4	0.213	0.148	0.457	0.230	-	0.124	0.191
C 5	0.330	0.112	0.363	0.334	0.117	-	0.286
C 6	0.062	0.305	0.650	0.041	0.200	0.306	-

4   Survival Analysis

Our analysis on users' roles has revealed that the level of users' engagement in an OHC is related to their posting behaviors on various types of social supports. The goal of conducting survival analysis in this section is to more systematically study social support factors related to users' engagement. In addition to users' posting behaviors, we also wanted to examine whether the exposure to different types of social support would impact a user's engagement. An individual may enter or exit a community not only based on his/her own expectation and behavior, but also based on the community's expectations and behaviors regarding this individual [21].

Our survival analysis was based on the Cox Proportional-Hazards Model [22,23], which assessed the importance of different independent variables on the "survival time" it takes for a specific event to occur. The hazard $h_i(t)$ represents the events occur to individual i at time t (defined as Equation-3),

$$h_i(t) = h_0(t) * exp\{\beta_1 x_{i1} + \beta_2 x_{i2} + \cdots + \beta_k x_{ik}\} \tag{3}$$

where the baseline hazard function $h_0(t)$ can be any function of time t as long as $h_0(t) > 0$. x_i and β represent independent variables and corresponding coefficients. Equation-3 can also be formulated as Equation-4, where the ratio of two individuals' hazard functions does not depend on time t.

$$\frac{h_i(t)}{h_j(t)} = exp\{\beta_1(x_{i1} - x_{j1}) + \cdots + \beta_k(x_{ik} - x_{jk})\} \tag{4}$$

With Maximum Likelihood Estimates (MLE), β can be estimated with regard to the hazard. $\beta_k = 0$ would indicate that independent variable x_k has no association with survival time; $\beta_k > 0$ means that independent variable x_k induces a higher hazard of event occurring, and vice versa. Correspondingly, $exp\{\beta_k\}$ is the hazard ratio of independent variable x_k.

Specifically for our analysis, an "event" refers to a user's cease of activities in the OHC (i.e., "leaving the OHC"). A user's survival time was measured by the difference between her/his last and first posts in the OHC. Here we assumed that a user had left this OHC if she/he had no post during the last 12 weeks in our dataset. For those who were still with the OHC during the last 12 weeks, their survival time was right-censored because they were still participating in this OHC.

Table 9 summarizes independent variables in our model. Values of these variables were based on users' activities within the first month of their online activities. Data was collected for 19,135 users whose time spans of activities exceeded one month. To reduce the impact of multi-collinearity, we calculated the correlation coefficients for every pair of independent variables. We then removed *TotalPost* and *NumThread* from the model, as they are strongly correlated with several other independent variables (with correlation coefficients greater than 0.8). Thus our full model for survival analysis included 11 independent variables.

Table 10 shows the results of the full model. Independent variables with hazard ratio less than 1 contribute positively to the "survival" (i.e., engagement) of users, whereas those with hazard ratio higher than 1 are considered "hazardous" to keep users in this OHC. For example, the hazard ratio of 0.907 for *COM* means that a user's "survival" rate after one month is 9.3% higher (100%-90.7%) if her number of companionship posts is one standard deviation higher than the average. Similarly, those who posted more to seek emotional support (*SES*) tended to stay with the OHC for longer. By contrast, those who sought and received more informational support (*SIS* and *RIS_D*) often left the OHC earlier. Besides the four, other independent variables are not significant predictors of users' time span of activities.

Table 9. Independent variables in survival analysis

Indep. Variables	Descriptions
TotalPost	The total number of posts a user has published
InitPost	The total number of threads a user initiates
NumThread	The number of threads a user contributed to (excluding those initiated by the user)
PES	The number of a user's posts that provided emotional support
PIS	The number of a user's posts that provided informational support
SES	The number of a user's posts that sought emotional support
SIS	The number of a user's posts that sought informational support
COM	The number of a user's posts that were related to companionship
RIS_D	Direct informational support received--the number of informational support posts a user received after initiating a support-seeking thread.
RES_D	Direct emotional support received--the number of emotional support posts a user received after initiating a support-seeking thread.
RIS_I	Indirect informational support received--the number of informational support posts a user was exposed to in threads that she/he did not initiate but contributed to.
RES_I	Indirect emotional support received--the number of emotional support posts a user was exposed to in threads that she/he did not initiate but contributed to.
RCOM	Companionship received--the number of companionship posts a user was exposed to in threads that she/he did not initiate but contributed to.

Note: for RIS_I, RES_I, and *RCOM*, we assumed that a user read others' replies that were posted within 7 days before the user's replies.

Table 10. Full model of survival analysis

Independent Variables	Hazard Ratio	Std. Err.
InitPost	0.990	0.0171
PES	1.015	0.0137
PIS	0.977	0.0162
SES	0.958***	0.0117
SIS	1.055***	0.0134
COM	0.907***	0.0131
RIS_D	1.048*	0.0192
RES_D	0.993	0.0137
RIS_I	1.040	0.0221
RES_I	0.970	0.0236
RCOM	0.968	0.0212

*:$p<0.05$, ***: $p<0.001$

To evaluate the robustness of the full model, we conducted the same analysis using backward sequential elimination [24]. Specifically, for the full Cox model with 11 independent variables, we removed the least significant variable in each iteration of the Cox model, until all independent variables left in the model were statistically significant. The four independent variables that were statistically significant in the full model were still significant and with similar hazard ratios after the last iteration of backward sequential elimination (shown in Table 11).

Table 11. Coefficients of 4 independent variables after backward sequential elimination

Independent Variables	Hazard Ratio	Std. Err.
SES	0.955***	0.0109
SIS	1.049***	0.0112
COM	0.906***	0.0122
RIS$_D$	1.032***	0.0103

***: p<0.001

5   Discussions

According to our survival analysis, those who started the first month of their online activities in the OHC with a lot of information seeking posts may not get engaged in the long run, even though they may also receive plenty of informational support as a result. This is in accordance with what a previous study found about informational support [17] and our analysis on users' roles in Section 3 (users in Cluster 3). In other words, informational support seekers have a higher chance of "churn" after they get the information they want from the community. This suggests that although community members have spent a lot of effort in providing informational support, as evidenced by the large number of *PIS* posts in Table 5, informational support does not seem to be the key to keep users engaged.

Conversely, those who were involved in companionship activities are more likely to stay. The positive effect of companionship on user engagement is even stronger than seeking emotional support, which was suggested to be a strong indicator of engagement by [17]. The exposure to companionship *RCOM* also has a hazard ratio below 1, although it is not statistically significant. The hazard ratios of both companionship-related independent variables indicate the importance of companionship. Similarly, in our user role analysis, community builders in Cluster 1 are very active. This is a very interesting finding—even though this is an OHC about cancer, it was the discussions of non-cancer-related issues (e.g., everyday family life and online games) that kept users engaged in the community. Recall that companionship includes discussions of offline events, sharing daily life stories that are more personal, and playing online games. We conjecture that companionship can strengthen the ties among users more than informational support that often lacks the personal touch, or emotional support, which can sometimes be generic and a mere formality (e.g., "I will pray for you", "Love you and Hug").

Another observation from the survival analysis is that none of the three independent variables for indirect support (*RIS$_I$, RES$_I$, and RCOM*) was statistically significant.

While it might be true that indirectly received support is not related to users' engage-ment, this may also be caused by our inaccurate measure of indirect support a user received. In our model, we assumed that a user received indirect support when she read a thread initiated by another user and other users' replies to the thread. This can be problematic: on one hand, we may underestimate the amount of support because we limited our calculation to threads a user replied to. In fact, a user can get indirect support from a thread without posting a reply. On the other hand, our approach can also overestimate such indirect support, because when posting to a long thread, a user may not have time to read all the previous replies, even though they were published within 7 days before the user's reply. Additional data of users' click streams will be needed to address this problem.

6   Conclusions and Future Work

This research analyzed users' behavioral patterns related to different types of social support and how such patterns are related to their engagement in an OHC. Using an OHC for breast cancer as a case study, we built classification models to detect the nature of social support in each post. After aggregating each user's posts, we grouped users based on their social support behavioral patterns and discovered seven different user roles in the OHC. Through comparisons between different roles and more sys-tematic survival analysis, we found that those with high level of engagement in the OHC are actively involved in companionship. In other words, sharing stories from personal daily life and activities that are not directly related to cancer are the key for keeping this community together. This is followed by seeking emotional support, which can also keep user engaged. On the other hand, simply seeking and receiving informational support makes a user vulnerable to churn.

The outcome of our study can shed light on the design and management of an OHC. For example, to keep an OHC active and sustainable, community managers may want to initiate and promote companionships activities, such as holiday plan dis-cussions, gardening tips, online scrabble games, offline gatherings, etc. Also, a thread/post recommender that leverages users' roles in the community can help profi-cient providers of certain support quickly find those who that are seeking such support. For future research, we would like to build a predictive model of user en-gagement based on our findings. Exploring whether a user's role changes over time would also be an interesting direction.

References

1. Fox, S.: The Social Life of Health Information, 2011. Pew Research Center's Internet & American Life Project (2011)
2. Chou, W.S., Hunt, Y.M., Beckjord, E.B., Moser, R.P., Hesse, B.W.: Social Media Use in the United States: Implications for Health Communication. J. Med. Internet Res. 11 (2009)
3. Kim, E., et al.: The process and effect of supportive message expression and reception in online breast cancer support groups. Psycho-Oncology 21, 531–540 (2012)
4. Rodgers, S., Chen, Q.: Internet Community Group Participation: Psychosocial Benefits for Women with Breast Cancer. Journal of Computer-Mediated Communication 10 (2005)

5. Dunkel-Schetter, C.: Social Support and Cancer: Findings Based on Patient Interviews and Their Implications. Journal of Social Issues 40, 77–98 (1984)
6. Qiu, B., Zhao, K., Mitra, P., Wu, D., Caragea, C., Yen, J., Greer, G.E., Portier, K.: Get Online Support, Feel Better – Sentiment Analysis and Dynamics in an Online Cancer Survivor Community. In: Privacy, Security, Risk and Trust (passat), Proceedings of the Third IEEE Third International Conference on Social Computing (SocialCom 2011), pp. 274–281 (2011)
7. Zhao, K., Yen, J., Greer, G., Qiu, B., Mitra, P., Portier, K.: Finding influential users of online health communities: a new metric based on sentiment influence. Journal of the American Medical Informatics Association: JAMIA (2014) (online first)
8. McClellan, W.M., Stanwyck, D.J., Anson, C.A.: Social support and subsequent mortality among patients with end-stage renal disease. JASN 4, 1028–1034 (1993)
9. Maloney-Krichmar, D., Preece, J.: A Multilevel Analysis of Sociability, Usability, and Community Dynamics in an Online Health Community. ACM Trans. Comput. 12, 201–232 (2005)
10. Idriss, S.Z., Kvedar, J.C., Watson, A.: The role of online support communities: Benefits of expanded social networks to patients with psoriasis. Arch. Dermatol. 145, 46–51 (2009)
11. Bambina, A.: Online social support: the interplay of social networks and computer-mediated communication. Cambria Press, Youngstown (2007)
12. Keating, D.M.: Spirituality and Support: A Descriptive Analysis of Online Social Support for Depression. J. Relig. Health 52, 1014–1028 (2013)
13. Krause, N.: Social Support, Stress, and Well-Being Among Older Adults. J. Gerontol. 41, 512–519 (1986)
14. Zhang, M., Yang, C.C., Gong, X.: Social Support and Exchange Patterns in an Online Smoking Cessa-tion Intervention Program. In: 2013 IEEE International Conference on Healthcare Informatics (ICHI), pp. 219–228 (2013)
15. Nambisan, P.: Information seeking and social support in online health communities: impact on patients' perceived empathy. J. Am. Med. Inform. Assoc. 18, 298–304 (2011)
16. Ahmed, O.H., Sullivan, S.J., Schneiders, A.G., Mccrory, P.: iSupport: do social networking sites have a role to play in concussion awareness? Disabil. Rehabil. 32, 1877–1883 (2010)
17. Wang, Y.-C., Kraut, R., Levine, J.M.: To stay or leave?: the relationship of emotional and informa-tional support to commitment in online health support groups. In: Proceedings of the ACM 2012 Conference on Computer Supported Cooperative Work, pp. 833–842 (2012)
18. Wilson, T., Wiebe, J., Hoffmann, P.: Recognizing Contextual Polarity in Phrase-level Sentiment Analysis. In: Proceedings of the Conference on Human Language Technology and Empirical Methods in Natural Language Processing, pp. 347–354 (2005)
19. Blei, D.M., Ng, A.Y., Jordan, M.I.: Latent Dirichlet Allocation. J. Mach. Learn. Res. 3, 993–1022 (2003)
20. Davies, D.L., Bouldin, D.W.: A Cluster Separation Measure. IEEE Transactions on Pattern Analysis and Machine Intelligence PAMI-1(2), 224–227 (1979)
21. Levine, J.M., Moreland, R.L.: Group Socialization: Theory and Research. European Review of Social Psychology 5, 305–336 (1994)
22. Cox, D.R.: Regression models and life tables. Journal of the Royal Statistical Society, Series B 34(2), 187–220 (1972)
23. Fox, J.: Cox proportional-hazards regression for survival data (2002),
http://socserv.mcmaster.ca/jfox/books/companion/appendix/Appendix-Cox-Regression.pdf (retrieved)
24. Cotter, S.F., Kreutz-Delgado, K., Rao, B.D.: Backward sequential elimination for sparse vector subset selection. Signal Processing 81, 1849–1864 (2001)

Doctor's Effort Influence on Online Reputation and Popularity

Xiaoxiao Liu[*], Xitong Guo, Hong Wu, and Doug Vogel

eHealth Research Institute, School of Management, Harbin Institute of Technology, China
{xiaoxiaoliuhit,xitongguo,hongwuhit,vogel.doug}@gmail.com

Abstract. This research examines why doctors participate in online activities and how they fully use online effort. We identify two dimensions of effort, i.e., online healthcare community function breadth (OHCFB), the number of different online functions used, and online healthcare community function depth (OHCFD), the degree of involvement with use of special online functions. We examine the effect of these two dimensions of online effort on doctor's online reputation and popularity and the impact of interaction between OHCFB and OHCFD. The study has three major findings: a) doctor's effort can increase their reputation and popularity, b) doctors with a low title have the potential to overcome shortcomings to increase popularity if they give special attention to a few select functions; however, doctors with a high title should try to expand the number of functions, and c) the interaction effect between OHCFB and OHCFD manifests differently across reputation and popularity.

Keywords: online healthcare community, effort, reputation, popularity.

1 Introduction

Healthcare is one of the most important aspects in people's life. With the rapid development of Internet technology, the online healthcare community has come into people's horizon. According to the Health Online 2013, the number of adults who use the Internet to search online health information has increased to 59% in the U.S. [1]. In addition, the Chinese government also has opened the medical market further and encourages doctors to serve patients through multiple channels [2].

With the rapid development of Web 2.0, the use of social media and its ability to promote the connection between patients and others is called "Health 2.0" [3]. Thus, online healthcare community is becoming one of the most important channels to promote medical service. Online healthcare communities provide doctors with many functions to help doctors provide better service. For example, through these communities, a registered doctor can write medical articles to help patients get more medical information. Further, a Q&A function can be opened by the doctor to solve patients' problems. Doctors use these functions with varying effort to achieve their goals. For patients, online healthcare community is a platform that they can search for health information, e.g., suggestions to help them recuperate.

Research has studied the benefits of online healthcare community from different perspectives [3]. McGeady, Kujala and Ilvonen [4] study information delivery between

---

[*] Corresponding author.

X. Zheng et al. (Eds.): ICSH 2014, LNCS 8549, pp. 111–126, 2014.

patients and doctors and discover that online community can increase quality of care due to increase the communication between patients and doctors. Sillence, Briggs, Harris and Fishwick [5] analyze whether patients trust online consultation or not. The Internet can affect people's decisions and similar experience can change the level of trust. Yang and Tan [6] believe that emotional support can help patients move to a healthier state and Kucukyazici, Verter and Mayo [7] argue that online healthcare community can provide information support for patients.

However, the benefits to patients from an online healthcare community can't be obtained without doctors' active participation. Therefore, it is important to study why doctors participate in online activities and how doctors make full use of their effort to achieve their goals. Doctors' active participation promotes improvement of their personal value through the quality and quantity of various functions provided by online healthcare community. Doctors who participate in the online communities want to spread reputation and word of mouth and achieve increased popularity.

Many online healthcare communities have provided quality and quantity rewards: giving more marks about one's reputation and displaying the volume of patients who know the doctors. However, little research has been done on why doctors participate in the online activities and how doctors make full use of their effort to achieve their goals. The object of this study is to analyze how the involvement of online effort impacts doctor's reputation and popularity using data collected from an online healthcare community. Our main research questions are:

- Does active participation (effort) in online healthcare community increase doctors' reputation and popularity?
- How can doctors make full use of effort to achieve their goals according to their personal information?

The rest of the paper is organized as follows. In section 2, we review and summarize literature on reputation, popularity and effort. This is followed by the presentation of our research hypotheses. Analysis is provided in section 3 and regression results are provided in section 4. The paper is discussed in section 5. Section 6 concludes the paper with future research directions.

2   Literature Review and Hypotheses

2.1   Reputation (quality) and Popularity (quantity)

Popularity and reputation are two common indexes to evaluate product image. They are the two dimensions of a brand. Popularity is the degree that a product is known by the public. It evaluates the product from the perspective of quantity. Reputation is the degree that the social public gives a positive evaluation to the product or service. It evaluates the product from the perspective of quality. Information cues such as brand names have effect on perceived quality, and a well-known brand name can be perceived as being of higher quality [8]. That is to say, a good product image can bring benefits to the sales of the product.

However, through the analysis of online search behavior, patients don't know doctor's detail information. First of all, they often want to know doctor's reputation (the evaluation that other patients make) and then make a choice to select doctors to consult, thus generating the popularity of the doctor. Based on the above content, we divide doctor's personal value into two aspects: quality and quantity. Quality means doctor's reputation and quantity means doctor's popularity.

2.2   Effort

Effort can be defined as "the amount of energy spent on an act per unit of time" [9], and the duration of time spent working and the intensity of work activities represent two important aspects of effort [10]. Based on the above content, we use the intensity of using online functions to measure doctor's online effort. Some empirical research has indicated that there is a positive relationship between effort and performance [11, 12]. In addition, employee's effort put into work can influence consumers' perception of service [13]. Then it increases frequency of visits and affects consumers' purchase attention because marketing efforts are likely to influence a positive sales transaction [14, 15]. This positive effect may lead to goods been browsed and bought frequently. Because online healthcare service belong to the service industry, we can assume that doctor's effort put into their work can affect patients' perception of service quality and their choice, which can affect patients willingness to appreciate the doctor's details further and the evaluation of patients for the doctor.

Because doctors promote their personal value by using various functions (See Table 1) provided by online healthcare community, we divide doctor's online effort into two aspects. Online Healthcare Community Function Breadth (OHCFB) refers to the number of functions, which are provided by online healthcare community and used by the doctor. It means that doctors expend energy to use a large variety of online healthcare community functions in their Internet work. Online Healthcare Community Function Depth (OHCFD) refers to the extent of experience that doctors have with using select online healthcare community functions. It captures the degree of experience with using online healthcare community functions. Table 2 is the description of different breadth and depth of effort.

Table 1. Functions for doctors provided in an online healthcare community

Function	Description
Online Q&A	This function allows patients to ask questions online (after the doctor opened the function) and can increase the interaction between doctors and patients.
Articles	This function allows doctors to write and publish medical articles and can help patients get more information, and also allows patients to append a message after the article.
Telephone consultation	This function allows patients to contact doctors by telephone consultation (after the doctor opened the function).
Patients community	This function allows doctors to create a community to help patients communicate with each other more conveniently, and get more information about the doctors.
Online appointment	This function allows patients to make an appointment with the doctor online (after the doctor opened the function).
Update outpatient services	This function allows doctors to update personal information, outpatient service, etc.

Table 2. Effort Distribution Patterns Across Online Healthcare Community Function

		Online Healthcare Community Function Depth (OHCFD)	
		Low	High
Online Healthcare Community Function Breadth (OHCFB)	Low	A doctor who put his(her) low effort into select functions	A doctor who put his(her) high effort into select functions
	High	A doctor who put his(her) low effort into many functions	A doctor who put his(her) high effort into many functions

A higher breadth of used functions suggests that the doctor puts more effort in using a large variety of services. However, a higher depth of used functions reflects that the doctor puts more effort in using select functions. Though doctors can use many functions to show their active participation to attract patients, they must put much effort in increasing the experience of using functions. Otherwise, the effectiveness of online effort may be impaired. Therefore, promoting reputation and popularity efficiently requires not only increasing the number of used functions, but also the involvement level of effort with using these functions. So, we argue that OHCFB and OHCFD complement each other in promoting reputation and popularity.

The difference between this paper and other works is that we conduct the study from the perspective of doctors and divide online effort into two dimensions to exposure why doctors participate in online healthcare community and how they fully use online effort.

Thus, we hypothesize that:

H1a. Greater breadth of online healthcare community functions that doctors use will be positively associated with doctors' popularity.

H1b. Greater depth of online healthcare community functions that doctors use will be positively associated with doctors' popularity.

H1c. Interaction between breadth and depth of online healthcare community functions that doctors use will be positively associated with doctors' popularity.

H2a. Greater breadth of online healthcare community functions that doctors use will be positively associated with doctors' reputation.

H2b. Greater depth of online healthcare community functions that doctors use will be positively associated with doctors' reputation.

H2c. Interaction between breadth and depth of online healthcare community functions that doctors use will be positively associated with doctors' reputation.

2.3   Doctor Title

Doctor title has two aspects: medical and education. Medical title includes resident doctor, attending doctor, associate chief physician and chief physician. Education title includes lecturer, associate professor and professional. However, every doctor has a medical title and it has no relationship with hospital level. But many doctors don't have an education title unless they belong to medical university-affiliated hospital. Therefore, patients may not care about the doctor's education title. Hence, this paper only analyses the moderating effect of medical title.

H3a. *The relationship between effort breadth and popularity is stronger for the doctor who has a high title than for those with a low title.*

H3b. *The relationship between effort depth and popularity is stronger for the doctor who has a low title than for those with a high title.*

H3c. *The relationship between effort breadth and reputation is stronger for the doctor who has a high title than for those with a low title.*

H3d. *The relationship between effort depth and reputation is stronger for the doctor who has a low title than for those with a high title.*

Fig. 1 is our research model.

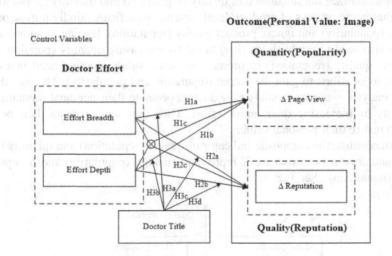

Fig. 1. Research model (⊗ is the interaction of effort breadth and effort depth)

3   Empirical Analyses

3.1   The Research Context

Our research context is Haodaifu Online (See Fig. 2), one of the most popular online healthcare communities. Several big companies have participated, such as Tencent, Sina, and Sohu. Allowing patients to search healthcare information and contact doctors as well as providing several functions for doctors to serve patients, Haodaifu is an active community to attract doctors and prospective patients. Launched in 2006, it already has nearly 3,235 hospitals and more than 323,732 doctors from 31 provinces. According to the statistics of the website, the number of page views per day is more than 3 million.

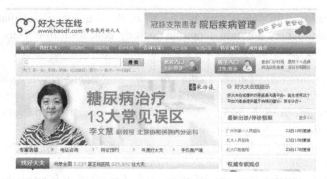

Fig. 2. Haodf.com home page (from March 2014)

Doctors can participate in Haodaifu to spread reputation and increase popularity. Many products face the imbalance of quality (reputation) and quantity (popularity). It means that in the process of product development, some firms blindly pursue product quantity (popularity) and ignore product quality (reputation), leading to an imbalance. Doctors also need to establish his (her) brand by increasing quantity (popularity) and enhancing quality (reputation) to promote personal value. Doctors need investment (referred to as effort) to gain the output (reputation and popularity). Through the following analysis, we want to study how doctors promote their personal reputation and popularity by increasing their online effort. Then they can promote their personal brand to realize their personal value.

We standardize the composite indicator of quality (reputation) and quantity (popularity), and draw a matrix where X represents quantity (popularity) and Y represents quality (reputation). (See Fig. 3)

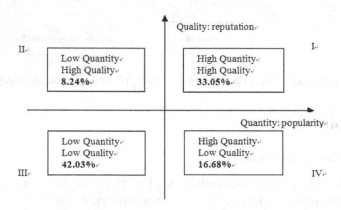

Fig. 3. Matrix of quality (reputation) and quantity (popularity)

According to the matrix, doctors distribute into four quadrants: high quantity and high quality (33.05%), low quantity and high quality (account for 8.24%), low quantity and low quality (42.03%) and high quantity and low quality (16.68%).

The first quadrant represents the strongest doctors; they attract most of the patients.

The second quadrant represents the most promising doctors; they have the most potential to develop.

The third quadrant represents the weakest doctors; they have the weakest effect on patients.

The fourth quadrant draws attention to the poorest received doctors; they leave a bad impression on patients.

There are close to half of the doctors in the third quadrant and doctors in the second and fourth quadrant total about 25%. These doctors are the people that don't balance their quality (reputation) and quantity (popularity) well. They should pay attention to their effort to enter the first quadrant to realize their personal value.

3.2   Data Collection

Data was collected from Haodf.com. We chose the disease of infertility as the research object and select the data in a one-month time span (December 2013 to January 2014). Then, from the doctors' own personal webpage, we collected the data for the number of letters of thanks, the number of gifts, and the number of votes and so on. We also collected doctors' personal information, e.g., gender, hospital level and title. The sample size for our study is 673 doctors. In sum, we collected the following data:

- The number of letters of thanks, gifts and votes the patients gave to the doctor.
- The gender, hospital level and city about the doctor's personal information.
- Information about the functions that the doctor is using.
- The number of patients who have browsed the doctor's homepage.

3.3   Variables

In order to test our hypotheses, we use the following variables.

Dependent Variable. The dependent variables in this study are doctor's online reputation and popularity. Reputation is the degree that the social public gives a positive evaluation to the doctor. It evaluates the doctor from the perspective of quality. Letters of thanks, gifts and votes in the website are given by patients who think the doctor help them. They are the evaluation given to the doctor. So, we use letters of thanks, gifts and votes to measure doctor's online reputation, and we use the following method to calculate the total reputation.

$$\Delta Rep = Z(\ln(\Delta Let + 1)) + Z(\ln(\Delta Gif + 1)) + Z(\ln(\Delta Vot + 1)) \tag{1}$$

Where

ΔRep represents the total reputation of the doctor that changed in 30 days; ΔLet represents the number of letters of thanks to the doctor that changed in 30 days; ΔGif represents the number of gifts to the doctor that changed in 30 days; ΔVot represents the number of the votes that doctors received from patients that changed in 30 days; Z(variable) means the variable is standardized in the paper.

Popularity is the level of awareness. The page views reflect the number of people who view the doctor's detailed information. We use the following method to calculate the total popularity.

$$\Delta Pop = \Delta Vie \tag{2}$$

Where

ΔPop represents the total popularity of the doctor that changed in 30 days; ΔVie represents page views of the doctor's home page that changed in 30 days.

Independent Variables. We select effort breadth and effort depth as the independent variables. We define $OHCFB$ as the number of functions that the doctor has used, and $OHCFD$ as the average degree of experience that the doctor has accumulated.

Computation of $OHCFB$

$$OHCFB_i = \sum_{j=1}^{N} B_{ij} \tag{3}$$

Where

B_{ij} indicates whether the doctor i use the online healthcare community function j, it takes the value of 0 or 1; N represents the number of online healthcare community functions offered by the website.

Computation of $OHCFD$

$$OHCFD_i = \frac{\sum_{j=1}^{N} \{Z(D_{ij}) \times B_{ij}\}}{\sum_{j=1}^{N} B_{ij}} \tag{4}$$

Where

B_{ij} indicates whether the doctor i use the online healthcare community function j, it takes the value of 0 or 1; N represents the number of online healthcare community functions offered by the website. D_{ij} represents the degree of experience that the doctor i accumulate in function j.

The following table is the value of effort breadth and depth.

Table 3. The Value of effort breadth and depth

Function	Breadth	Depth
Function 1	article	the number of articles
Function 2	patients community	the number of communities that the doctor has opened
Function 3	online consultation	the average amount of response in two weeks

Control Variables. We control for other factors that may impact doctor's reputation and popularity, such as hospital level and the regional economy where the hospital is in. China divides hospitals into three levels and each level has A, B and C standards. Because of different infrastructure and staff, patients may tend to know the doctors who work in high level hospitals. In the same way, the regional economy has the same effect on patients' decision. In addition, doctors' gender may be a factor in patients' choice. The doctor's owned reputation also affects doctor's popularity. We use the number of letters of thanks (*Olet*), gifts (*Ogif*) and votes (*Ovot*) that the doctor have received to represent the doctor's owned reputation.

$$Orep = Z(\ln(Olet + 1)) + Z(\ln(Ogif + 1)) + Z(\ln(Ovot)) \tag{5}$$

Where

Orep represents the reputation that the doctor has received; *Olet* represents the number of letters of thanks that the doctor has received; *Ogif* represents the number of gift that the doctor has received; *Ovot* represents the number of the votes that the doctor has received.

Thus, we control the hospital level (*Hle*), the region economy (*Eco*), the doctors' gender (*Gender*) and the doctors' owned reputation (*Orep*). We also control doctor's education title (*Etitdummy$_1$* and *Etitdummy$_2$*).

3.4 Analysis Method

We use ordinary least squares regression and hierarchical regression to test our hypotheses and formulate the following empirical model.

$$
\begin{aligned}
\ln \Delta Pop = {} & \beta_0 + \beta_1 \ln OHCFB + \beta_2 OHCFD + \beta_3 \ln OHCFB \times OHCFD \\
& + \beta_4 \sum_{i=1,2} \ln OHCFB \times Mtitdummy_i + \beta_5 \sum_{i=1,2} OHCFD \times Mtitdummy_i \\
& + \beta_6 Hle + \beta_7 \ln Eco + \beta_8 Gender + \beta_9 Etitdummy_1 + \beta_{10} Etitdummy_2 \\
& + \beta_{11} Mtitdummy_1 + \beta_{12} Mtitdummy_2 + \beta_{13} Orep
\end{aligned}
\tag{6}
$$

$$
\begin{aligned}
\ln \Delta Rep = {} & \beta_0 + \beta_1 \ln OHCFB + \beta_2 OHCFD + \beta_3 \ln OHCFB \times OHCFD \\
& + \beta_4 \sum_{i=1,2} \ln OHCFB \times Mtitdummy_i + \beta_5 \sum_{i=1,2} OHCFD \times Mtitdummy_i \\
& + \beta_6 Hle + \beta_7 \ln Eco + \beta_8 Gender + \beta_9 Etitdummy_1 + \beta_{10} Etitdummy_2 \\
& + \beta_{11} Mtitdummy_1 + \beta_{12} Mtitdummy_2
\end{aligned}
\tag{7}
$$

4   Results

We report the summary statistics of our major variables in Table 4 and correlations between variables in Table 5.

Table 6 and Table 7 provide the results of the estimations. Model 1, Table 6 and Model 1, Table 7 analyze the effect of the control variables, whereas others contain the results with the control and predictor variables.

The results for Model 2, Table 6, indicate a positive and significant coefficient on OCHFB and OCHFD, which represents the popularity gains from online effort (Breadth regression coefficient=0.304, $p<0.01$ and depth regression coefficient=0.332, $p<0.01$) as hypothesized, thus H1a and H1b are supported. This result indicates that for doctor's popularity, breadth and depth of doctor's online effort are associated with higher popularity. H2a and H2b predict that the breadth and depth of online effort will be associated with higher doctor's reputation. The results for Model 2, Table 7, indicate that OCHFD has a positive and significant effect on reputation (Regression coefficient=0.443, $p<0.01$), as predicted by H2b. However, contrary to the predication in H2a, breadth of doctors' effort has no significant effect on reputation (Model 2, Table 7, regression coefficient=-0.073, $p>0.1$). Thus, H2a is not supported.

Now, we analyze the interaction between OHCFB and OCHFD. The negative and significant coefficient on $lnOHCFB \times OHCFD_{pop}$ (Model 3, Table 6, Regression coefficient=-0.092, $p<0.01$) indicates that OCHFB and OCHFD are substitutive for popularity. Taken together, these results (Table 6) suggest that, for popularity, the breadth and depth of doctor's online effort are sufficient by themselves for increasing popularity, thus H1c is not supported. However, for reputation, the coefficient on $lnOHCFB \times OHCFD_{rep}$ is positive and significant (Model 3, Table 7, Regression coefficient=0.083, $p<0.1$), and it is indicative of the presence of positive interaction between online healthcare community functions breadth (OHCFB) and online healthcare community functions depth (OCHFD), as predicted by H2c. Taken together, these results (Table 7) indicate that effort breadth affects the relationship between effort depth and reputation i.e., the higher the breadth, the stronger the relationship.

Then we test the moderating of medical title. We first define the medical title, $Mtitdummy_i$, as a dummy variable. $Mtitdummy_1$ takes the value of 1 if the title is associate chief physician and $Mtitdummy_2$ takes the value of 1 if the title is chief physician and the other is attending doctor. In model 4, Table 6, medical title has no relationship with popularity. Model 5, Table 6, gives the results of the interaction between $Mtitdummy_1$ and OHCFB and the interaction between $Mtitdummy_2$ and OHCFD. Results show that medical title is a pure moderator, indicating that the relationship between effort and popularity is contingent upon doctor title. Thus hypotheses 3a and 3b are supported ($lnOHCFB \times Mtitdummy_1$ regression coefficient=0.132, $p<0.01$; $lnOHCFB \times Mtitdummy_2$ regression coefficient=0.095, $p<0.05$; $OHCFD \times Mtitdummy_1$ regression coefficient=-0.126, $p<0.01$; $OHCFD \times Mtitdummy_2$ regression coefficient=-0.144, $p<0.05$). The results reveal preliminary that the popularity of the doctor who has a high title will increase faster than the doctor who has a low title if they put their effort into breadth. However, the doctor who has a low title will increase faster than the doctor who has a high title if they put their effort into depth. More research is needed to test the moderating effect.

Model 5, Table 7, shows that the medical title is not a moderator ($lnOHCFB \times Mtitdummy_1$ regression coefficient=0.026, p>0.1; $lnOHCFB \times Mtitdummy_2$ regression coefficient=-0.077, p>0.1; $OHCFD \times Mtitdummy_1$ regression coefficient=0.031, p>0.1; $OHCFD \times Mtitdummy_2$ regression coefficient=0.132, p>0.1). Thus hypotheses 3c and 3d are not supported.

The hypotheses test results from the data are summarized in Table 8 and Fig.5.

Table 4. Summary statistics

Variables	Mean	Std. Dev.	Minimum	Maximum
Hle	2.85	0.511	0	3
Eco	8185.418474	6137.9062149	234.5000	19195.6000
Gender	0.29	0.453	0	1
$Etitdummy_1$	0.18	0.388	0	1
$Etitdummy_2$	0.28	0.447	0	1
Orep	1.928287	2.9765331	-2.6701	11.2635
$Mtitdummy_1$	0.37	0.483	0	1
$Mtitdummy_2$	0.48	0.500	0	1
OHCFB	2.34	0.801	1	3
OHCFD	0.280539	0.7951950	-0.6919	3.6492
ΔRep	0.163986	2.5040897	-1.1482	16.1552
ΔPop	32324.87	63344.321	60	908456

Table 5. Correlation table

	1	2	3	4	5	6	7	8	9	10	11	12
Hle	1	0.068	0.036	0.062	0.094	0.094	-0.025	0.072	0.007	-0.027	0.074	0.008
lnEco	0.068	1	0.009	0.044	0.019	0.376	-0.007	0.014	0.075	0.138	0.219	0.246
Gender	0.036	0.009	1	-0.043	0.085	0.150	-0.028	0.016	0.156	0.248	0.088	0.186
$Etitdummy_1$	0.062	0.044	-0.043	1	-0.294	0.081	0.349	-0.197	-0.023	0.064	0.013	0.070
$Etitdummy_2$	0.094	0.019	0.085	-0.294	1	0.192	-0.455	0.612	0.040	0.088	0.094	0.102
Orep	0.094	0.376	0.150	0.081	0.192	1	-0.006	0.177	0.478	0.642	0.552	0.798
$Mtitdummy_1$	-0.025	-0.007	-0.028	0.349	-0.455	-0.006	1	-0.731	-0.006	-0.009	-0.011	-0.013
$Mtitdummy_2$	0.072	0.014	0.016	-0.197	0.612	0.177	-0.731	1	0.025	0.092	0.086	0.119
lnOHCFB	0.007	0.075	0.156	-0.023	0.040	0.478	-0.006	0.025	1	0.647	0.221	0.725
OHCFD	-0.027	0.138	0.248	0.064	0.088	0.642	-0.009	0.092	0.647	1	0.413	0.808
ΔRep	0.074	0.219	0.088	0.013	0.094	0.552	0.011	0.086	0.221	0.413	1	0.429
$ln\Delta Pop$	0.008	0.246	0.186	0.070	0.102	0.798	-0.013	0.119	0.725	0.808	0.429	1

lnOHCFB and OHCFD are standardized.

Table 6. Regression coefficients and model summary statistics for the test of popularity

Control and Independent variables	Dependent variable is $\ln\Delta Pop$				
	Model 1	Model 2	Model 3	Model 4	Model 5
Hle	-0.053**	-0.026	-0.023	-0.023	-0.021
lnEco	-0.075***	0.007	0.002	0.001	0.000
Gender	0.072***	-0.007	0.000	0.000	-0.004
Etitdummy$_1$	-0.014	0.011	0.006	0.011	0.017
Etitdummy$_2$	-0.067***	-0.019	-0.022	-0.034	-0.034
Orep	0.819***	0.445***	0.456***	0.459***	0.458***
lnOHCFB		0.304***	0.237***	0.237***	0.099*
OHCFD		0.332***	0.397***	0.395***	0.570***
lnOHCFB×OHCFD$_{pop}$			-0.092***	-0.092***	-0.087***
Mtitdummy$_1$				-0.027	-0.058**
Mtitdummy$_2$				0.002	-0.016
Mtitdumy$_1$×lnOHCFB					0.132***
Mtitdumy$_2$×lnOHCFB					0.095**
Mtitdummy$_1$×OHCFD					-0.126***
Mtitdummy$_2$×OHCFD					-0.144**
R-square	0.633	0.831	0.835	0.836	0.839
Adjusted R-Square	0.630	0.829	0.833	0.833	0.836
F-test (n=673)	191.561***	406.836***	373.890***	306.309***	229.051***
ΔF-test		386.820***	19.524***	1.196	3.557***

*   indicates $p<0.1$
**   Indicates $p<0.05$
*** Indicates $p<0.01$

Table 7. Regression coefficients and model summary statistics for the test of reputation

Control and Independent variables	Dependent variable is ΔRep				
	Model 1	Model 2	Model 3	Model 4	Model 5
Hle	0.042	0.067*	0.063*	0.062*	0.066*
lnEco	0.219***	0.173***	0.174***	0.175***	0.177***
Gender	0.081**	-0.017	-0.022	-0.021	-0.021
Etitdummy$_1$	0.029	-0.012	-0.008	-0.021	-0.016
Etitdummy$_2$	0.065	0.029	0.031	0.027	0.025
lnOHCFB		-0.073	-0.014	-0.013	0.032
OHCFD		0.443***	0.379***	0.377***	0.258*
lnOHCFB×OHCFD$_{rep}$			0.083*	0.081*	0.086*
Mtitdummy$_1$				0.072	0.067
Mtitdummy$_2$				0.055	0.059
Mtitdummy$_1$×lnOHCFB					0.026
Mtitdummy$_2$×lnOHCFB					-0.077
Mtitdummy$_1$×OHCFD					0.031
Mtitdummy$_2$×OHCFD					0.132
R-square	0.065	0.211	0.215	0.217	0.221
Adjusted R-Square	0.58	0.203	0.206	0.206	0.204
F-test (n=673)	9.252***	25.459***	22.779***	18.372***	13.318***
ΔF-test		61.762***	3.383*	0.800	0.751

*   Indicates $p<0.1$
**   Indicates $p<0.05$
*** Indicates $p<0.01$

Table 8. Summary hypotheses test results

Hypotheses	Supported?
H1a. Greater breadth of online healthcare community functions that doctors use will be positively associated with doctors' popularity.	Yes
H1b. Greater depth of online healthcare community functions that doctors use will be positively associated with doctors' popularity.	Yes
H1c. Interaction between breadth and depth of online healthcare community functions that doctors use will be positively associated with doctors' popularity.	No
H2a. Greater breadth of online healthcare community functions that doctors use will be positively associated with doctors' reputation.	No
H2b. Greater depth of online healthcare community functions that doctors use will be positively associated with doctors' reputation.	Yes
H2c. Interaction between breadth and depth of online healthcare community functions that doctors use will be positively associated with doctors' reputation.	Yes
H3a: The relationship between effort breadth and popularity is stronger for the doctor who has a high title than for those with a low title.	Yes
H3b: The relationship between effort depth and popularity is stronger for the doctor who has a low title than for those with a high title.	Yes
H3c: The relationship between effort breadth and reputation is stronger for the doctor who has a high title than for those with a low title.	No
H3d: The relationship between effort depth and reputation is stronger for the doctor who has a low title than for those with a high title.	No

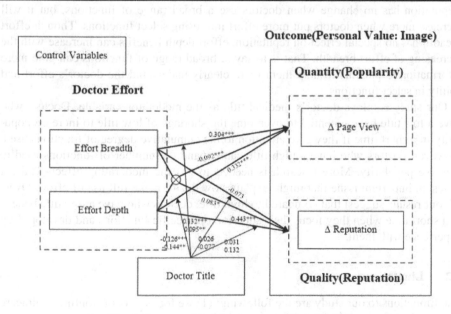

Fig. 4. Summary hypotheses test results in Model

5   Discussion

In this research, we examined the impact on reputation and popularity of effort that doctors put into online healthcare communities. Specifically, we test the reputation and popularity impacts of two dimensions of doctor's online effort, OHCFB and OHCFD. OHCFB measures the number of functions which are provided by an online healthcare community and used by the doctor, and OHCFD refers to the extent of experience that doctors have using select online healthcare community functions. Besides examining the independent impacts of OHCFB and OHCFD, we also examined the interaction between OHCFB and OHCFD. In addition, we tested the moderating effect of doctor's medical title.

5.1   Key Findings

Our empirical analysis uses data from 673 doctors. The results indicate the difference in the impacts of online healthcare community function breadth (OHCFB) and depth (OHCFD) across reputation and popularity. Popularity increased when doctors use more online functions or put more effort into select functions. But there are overlapping functionalities in attracting patients to view the doctor's home page to get more details by the breadth and depth of the effort. That is to say, a broad range of functions and a high degree of experience of using select functions are overlapping in increasing popularity. However, more research is needed to test the substitutive effect. Reputation has no change when doctors use a broad range of functions, but it will increase more when doctors put more effort into using select functions. Though effort breadth has no special effect on reputation, effort depth benefits can increase with the increasing of effort breadth. That is to say, a broad range of functions can give more information to patients to help them more clearly understand the doctor's effort and ability in select functions.

Our study employs doctor's medical title as the moderator variable. Doctors who have a low title have potential to overcome the shortage of low title to increase popularity in a short time if they give attention to the cumulative degree of functions used. However, doctors who have a high title can expand the number of functions used to increase popularity. More research is needed to test the moderating effect. Thus, it raises an important issue that might explain how doctor make full use of effort. Overall, our results suggest that compared to high title, doctors who have a low title benefit in a short time when they focus their attention on specific functions and develop deep experience with them.

5.2   Limitations

The limitations to our study are the following: (1) we focus only one online healthcare community because it is one of the most popularity communities. Different communities provide different functions for doctors. Also, the size of the community may influence the number and style of functions. Investigation is needed as to whether our findings can be generalized to other communities. (2) There are many functions for doctors provided in the online healthcare community, and we choose the major functions to test the model. Future research should relax this assumption. (3) Though we control the variables that can influence popularity and reputation, other influencing factor such as price, off-line effort, etc. may influence doctor's online popularity and reputation. Future research should include these factors. (4) Finally, the research is conducted in China and may not generalize to other cultures.

5.3 Directions for Future Research

Doctors facing different diseases may have different motivations to use the functions. In addition, the number of patients with different diseases (acute or chronic disease, etc.) may influence the way to increase doctor's reputation and popularity. Therefore, in future research, we can use different diseases to test the model and compare results. What's more, relevant avenues for future research are available in terms of different styles of online communities.

6   Conclusions

Because we control doctors' other information such as hospital level, the finding that doctor's online effort is positively related to doctor's online popularity and reputation answers the first research question. The two dimension of active participation (effort) can both increase doctors popularity, but their interaction may decrease the popularity because of the overlapping functionalities in breadth and depth of effort. Though increasing the number of functions used has no direct effect on doctor's reputation, it can influence the relationship between depth and reputation. Cumulative effort depth benefits can increase via increasing effort breadth. These results can explain why doctor participate in online healthcare community and help explain how they can make full use of effort (the second research question). Though doctors' objective information can affect doctor's popularity and reputation, they also can increase popularity and reputation through their online effort

The results regarding the moderation of doctor's medical title can explain how doctor take full use of effort. The results show that doctors with a low title have the potential to cover the shortage of low title to increase popularity in a short time if they pay attention to the cumulative degree of functions that used. However, doctors who have a high title can expand the number of functions used to increase popularity. That is to say, doctors who have a low title benefit in a short time when they focus their attention on specific functions and develop deep experience with them.

References

1. Fox, S., Duggan, M.: Health Online 2013, Health (2013)
2. China Released the Price of the Non-Public Hospital and Encourage Social do Medical, http://www.mzyfz.com/cms/pufazhuanlan/pufazhongxin/pufahuodong/html/1173/2014-04-09/content-993237.html

3. Ba, S., Wang, L.: Digital Health Communities: The Effect of Their Motivation Mechanisms. Decision Support Systems 55, 941–947 (2013)
4. McGeady, D., Kujala, J., Ilvonen, K.: The Impact of Patient–Physician Web Messaging on Healthcare Service Provision. International Journal of Medical Informatics 77, 17–23 (2008)
5. Sillence, E., Briggs, P., Harris, P.R., Fishwick, L.: How Do Patients Evaluate and Make Use of Online Health Information? Social Science & Medicine 64, 1853–1862 (2007)
6. Yang, L., Tan, Y.: Feeling Blue So Going Online: An Empirical Study on Effectiveness of Virtual Social Networking. In: Workshop on Health IT and Economics (2010)
7. Kucukyazici, B., Verter, V., Mayo, N.E.: An Analytical Framework for Designing Community-Based Care for Chronic Diseases. Production and Operations Management 20, 474–488 (2011)
8. Wall, M., Liefeld, J., Heslop, L.A.: Impact of Country-of-Origin Cues on Consumer Judgments in Multicue Situations: a Covariance Analysis. Journal of the Academy of Marketing Science 19, 105–113 (1991)
9. Naylor, J.C., Pritchard, R.D., Ilgen, D.R.: A Theory of Behavior in Organizations. Academic Press, New York (1980)
10. Campbell, J.P., Pritchard, R.D.: Motivation Theory in Industrial and Organizational Psychology. In: Handbook of Industrial and Organizational Psychology, vol. 1, pp. 63–130 (1983)
11. Brown, S.P., Peterson, R.A.: The Effect of Effort on Sales Performance and Job Satisfaction. The Journal of Marketing, 70–80 (1994)
12. Mengüç, B.: Evidence for Turkish Industrial Salespeople: Testing the Applicability of a Conceptual Model for the Effect of Effort on Sales Performance and Job Satisfaction. European Journal of Marketing 30, 33–51 (1996)
13. Bitner, M.J., Booms, B.H., Mohr, L.A.: Critical Service Encounters: The Employee's Viewpoint. Journal of Marketing 58, 95–106 (1994)
14. McClean, E., Collins, C.J.: High-Commitment HR Practices, Employee Effort, and Firm Performance: Investigating the Effects of HR Practices Across Employee Groups within Professional Services Firms. Human Resource Management 50, 341–363 (2011)
15. Borucki, C.C., Burke, M.J.: An Examination of Service-Related Antecedents to Retail Store Performance. Journal of Organizational Behavior 20, 943–962 (1999)

Extended Abstract: Study on the Design for Consumer Health Knowledge Organization System in China

Li Hou

Institute of Medical Information, Chinese Academy of Medical Sciences,
Beijing, China, 100020
hou.li@imicams.ac.cn

Objective: In order to bridge the "knowledge gap" between the technical terms used by healthcare professionals and the health terms by consumers, this paper designs a knowledge representation method to organize various health concepts and terms which can be understanding by general public in China.

Background and Significance: With the development of information technology, it is becoming increasingly evident that more and more consumers are using the Internet to seek medical or health related information. According to the seventh national reading survey data subcontinent Chinese Institute of Publishing Science in 2009 showed that 83%of Chinese people choose digital reading [1], which is 83.4% of the public access to health information through search engines. With the rapid development of biomedical, there are more and more professional medical terms in biomedical field, such as "acquired immunodeficiency syndrome", which is unfamiliar term to public. If the website designer developing health knowledge service platform use such term to describe disease or organize health knowledge, it is difficult for public to understand, or to seek health knowledge which they need. In order to build a bridge between the medical professional terms with the understanding of public and the vocabulary used by public, and to enhance the ability of the medical information institute for public health. It is necessary to construct consumer health vocabulary, and how to organize various expression of medical terms is the key step.

Knowledge organization system covers a variety of organizational information framework, such as terminology, dictionary, classification and ontology [2, 3], knowledge organization system includes a variety of properties which make every term has clearer semantic, some standardized biomedical terminology, such as SNOMED CT, ICD, are used to be the exchange standards in different Clinical Information System. But this kind of terminology is still professional one, which cannot be used to organize consumer health vocabulary. It is important to design the framework of consumer health knowledge organization system, which is helpful for public to reading and understanding healthcare knowledge.

Method: There are variety type of health knowledge which general public concerns, according to the content there are such types: diseases, drugs, symptoms, diagnostic tests, hospitals, doctors, nutrition and health information[4].We propose to narrow down the research object, and focus on diseases and pharmaceuticals data. We

X. Zheng et al. (Eds.): ICSH 2014, LNCS 8549, pp. 127–129, 2014.

develop a knowledge representation method for diseases and pharmaceuticals data based on the framework of concept and attribute of concept.

Design Idea: A three-step workflow is designed to regulate the concept of diseases and pharmaceuticals which public concerns, and normalize the different forms of expression on one same concept. First, the concept of disease and pharmaceutical is extracted, which is described concept C. Second, we make use of concept to organize other relevant terminology, and add attribute for every concept denoted by A^c, so we can form the semantic network of health data, the method can be described as: K = {C, A^c }. Thirdly, an experiment is conducted. Specific steps are as follows:

Design Concept Table and Descriptive Method: The first step is to define the standard of different types of health concepts and terminology. In principle, the concept will be determined in accordance with international accepted standards, if there is no international accepted standard, we adopt the industry standard to define concepts and terminology. For disease, the vocabularies which tree number are under C21 in Medical Subject Headings are taken as concept, the other health vocabularies from scientific material are taken as term. For pharmaceutical, we take the generic medicament in "chinese pharmacopoeia" as concept, take the trade name as term. The second step is to define the naming rules on describing different entities of diseases and pharmaceuticals. The third step is to define every elements in Concept Table, including the meaning of elements and elements' abbreviation. What element refer to is the uniquely identifies, language, source, source table, the term name, the concept name, note, tree number and etc.

Design Attribute Table and Descriptive Method: Attribute is to describe the concept, additional information about the atoms or the relationship, which can be used for many purposes. Description of the attributes table may be different in different sources, referred to as $A^C = \{a_1, a_2, a_3 .... a_n\}$. What attribute refer to is unique identifier for term, unique identifier for string, unique identifier for attribute, attribute name, abbreviated source name, source asserted attribute identifier and etc.

Conduct Experiment: We extract the Subject Headings of disease in CMeSH, generic medicament in "Chinese Pharmacopoeia", and then select 1,077 disease name that consumer concern mostly as the concept, and select 1,267 generic medicament as concept of pharmaceutical, and then crawl relative disease name in science material and trade name in SFDA, map the 1,077 disease name to relative disease name in science material, map 1,267 generic medicament to trade name in SFDA. Lastly, we generate Concept Table and Attribute Table, and entry its unique value for every disease and pharmaceutical concept on the basis of the designing scheme.

Result: In this study, we attempt to design one knowledge representation method to organize various medical concepts and terms, we achieve this goal through two table, one is Concept Table, the another is Attribute of Concept Table. We map the common terms to the professional concepts by the synonymy relationship in CMeSH. As a result, we construct one consumer health knowledge organization system including 1,077 concepts of disease and 25,704 terms of disease, and 1,267 concepts of pharmaceutical, 16,180 terms of pharmaceutical. This work is an initial exploration, there is a long way to go for us to construct one thorough consumer health knowledge organization system.

References

[1] Peng, B.: Chinese Institute of Publishing Science "Sixth National Reading Survey" results released (2014), http://book.people.com.cn/GB/69839/120524/120531/14451149.html
[2] Dos Reis, J.C., Pruski, C., Da Silveira, M., Reynaud-Delaître, C.: Understanding semantic mapping evolution by observing changes in biomedical ontologies. Journal of Biomedical Informatics 25, 1532–1546 (2013)
[3] Hodge, G.: Systems of knowledge organization for digital libraries: beyond traditional authority files, pp. 5–6. Council on Library and Information Resources, Washington, DC (2000), http://old.diglib.org/pubs/dlf090/dlf090.pdf
[4] Li, D.: Medical Information Analyze, p. 24. People's Medical Publishing House, Beijing (2009)

Trend and Network Analysis of Common Eligibility Features for Cancer Trials in ClinicalTrials.gov

Chunhua Weng[1], Anil Yaman[2], Kuo Lin[1], and Zhe He[1]

[1] Department of Biomedical Informatics, Columbia University, New York City, USA
[2] Department of Computer Science, The City College of New York, New York City, USA
{cw2384,kl2734,zh2132}@columbia.edu, anilyaman00@gmail.com

Abstract. ClinicalTrials.gov has been archiving clinical trials since 1999, with > 165,000 trials at present. It is a valuable but relatively untapped resource for understanding trial design patterns and acquiring reusable trial design knowledge. We extracted common eligibility features using an unsupervised tag-mining method and mined their temporal usage patterns in clinical trials on various cancers. We then employed trend and network analysis to investigate two questions: (1) what eligibility features are frequently used to select patients for clinical trials within one cancer or across multiple cancers; and (2) what are the trends in eligibility feature adoption or discontinuation across cancer research domains? Our results showed that each cancer domain reuses a small set of eligibility features frequently for selecting cancer trial patients and some features are shared across different cancers, with value range adjustments for numerical measures. We discuss the implications for facilitating community-based clinical research knowledge sharing and reuse.

Keywords: Clinical Trials, Patient Selection, Knowledge Management.

1 Introduction

Knowledge management and standards-based clinical research design are two related tasks of high priority for the field of clinical research informatics since its inception. One type of clinical research, the randomized controlled trial, has long been accepted as the gold standard for generating high-quality medical evidence. Therefore, much effort has been devoted to developing formal representations for clinical trial protocols [1-5], clinical trial eligibility criteria [6, 7], or common data elements for clinical trial data collection [8-10]. Most of these efforts have resulted in ontologies or expert systems for supporting computational reuse of clinical trial eligibility criteria. However, due to the lack of interoperability among such ontologies or standards [11-13] and the high cost of text knowledge engineering for clinical research protocols, there has been limited adoption of these methods by the clinical research community for improving the computability of new clinical trial designs, which are usually written as lengthy, free-text paper documents.

Meanwhile, studies have also revealed the great need of the clinical research community for clinical research knowledge reuse [14, 15], as reflected by the fact that eligibility criteria texts for patient selection are often similar, and sometimes identical,

X. Zheng et al. (Eds.): ICSH 2014, LNCS 8549, pp. 130–141, 2014.

across different studies within the same disease domain or across different disease domains [15, 16]. Little is known about knowledge reuse patterns in clinical trial designs for patient selection, either within or across diseases, but such knowledge could potentially inform the construction of valuable trial design knowledge bases that address clinical researchers' needs for knowledge reuse. Moreover, the availability of ClinicalTrials.gov [17], the largest public clinical trial repository with over 165,000 trials for thousands of diseases as of April 2014, presents a valuable opportunity for using Big Data analytics to discover eligibility criteria knowledge reuse patterns from clinical trial summary text.

This paper reports the results of a preliminary attempt to analyze such patterns. Using cancer clinical trial eligibility criteria as an example, we employed network and trend analysis to address these two research questions: (1) what eligibility features are frequently used to select patients for clinical trials of one cancer type or across multiple cancer types; (2) what are the temporal patterns in adopting or rejecting frequently used eligibility features? We then discuss the implications for supporting knowledge reuse and sharing for clinical trial eligibility criteria designs in the future.

2   Methods

2.1   Selecting an Example Problem Domain: Cancer

Entering a disease name in the "Condition" field on the online search form provided by ClinicalTrials.gov can retrieve all clinical trial summaries for a specific medical condition. Given the global priority of cancer research, we decided to focus on clinical trial eligibility criteria for all cancers. Therefore, we retrieved and downloaded all the eligibility criteria text and information about their cancer types.

2.2   Mining Common Eligibility Features (CEFs) from Text

On ClinicalTrials.gov, all clinical trial eligibility criteria are stored and presented as unstructured text. We applied an unsupervised tag mining method [18] to extract discrete concepts from eligibility criteria text. The text was processed to remove special characters and punctuation and to build all the possible n-grams (i.e., continuous subsequences of n words). N-grams composed of only English stop words or irrelevant grammatical structures were removed. Each n-gram was matched against the Unified Medical Language System (UMLS)[19] Metathesaurus and retained only if at least one of its substrings was a recognizable UMLS concept. Moreover, we considered only those UMLS concepts appearing in semantic categories most relevant to the clinical trial domain. For example, "*malignancy within the past 5 years*" would be considered a valid n-gram because at least one word, "*malignancy*", was present in the part of the UMLS lexicon considered, even if the entire sentence were not. Each n-gram term found in the UMLS lexicon was also normalized according to its preferred Concept Unique Identifier (CUI). Using the CUIs increased the density of concepts and enabled the handling of synonyms, since similar concepts are aligned to the same preferred term by the UMLS specification (e.g., "*atrial fibrillation*" and "*auricular fibrillation*" are both mapped to "*atrial fibrillation*"). This allowed identifying semantically unique eligibility features. Since each CUI may be mapped to more than one UMLS semantic type, we also assigned to each n-gram a distinctive UMLS semantic type by performing semantic type disambiguation using previously defined semantic preference rules [20]. After this process, each clinical trial's eligibility criteria were summarized by a set of UMLS CUI-based n-grams representing the criteria's relevant features. On this basis, we retained the n-grams appearing in at least 20% of all cancer trials and considered them common eligibility features (CEFs).

2.3   Trend Pattern Generation for CEFs and Cancers Pairs, Respectively

We analyzed the pairwise trend similarity between CEFs. A CEF's occurrences over the 15 years formed a vector. We used the correlation coefficient significance test [21] to measure the correlation between any two vectors of the same length (e.g., length = 15 for CEFs) as follows:

$$\text{Cor(X, Y)} = \frac{\sum_{i=1}^{n}(x_i - \overline{x})(y_i - \overline{y})}{\sqrt{\sum_{i=1}^{n}(x_i - \overline{x})}\sqrt{\sum_{i=1}^{n}(y_i - \overline{y})}}$$

The CEFs that occur in less than three years were excluded because their temporal patterns were meaningless. The remaining CEFs' occurrences were normalized. We picked a P-value of 0.001 after preliminary experiments so that we only allowed 0.1% of chance for the identified correlation to be wrong. Using this P-value, according to the Correlation Coefficient Significance table, by using a degree of freedom of 13 since the length of each vector is 15, a significant relationship should have its correlation coefficient greater than 0.7603.

After identifying significant relationships in CEF pairs, we developed a temporal pattern matching method to automatically identify correlated CEF pairs based on their frequency changes in the 15 years. We divided the 15-year time interval into 14 consecutive subintervals. For each interval spanning two consecutive years (e.g., 2008-2009) for a certain CEF, we labeled it increasing, decreasing, or stable. We arrived at the temporal pattern for a CEF by concatenating the patterns in all 14 intervals.

To best match the real pattern of CEFs' frequencies, after manual test, we assigned each interval a specific category as follows: if a CEF's frequency in year (n+1) was 120% that of year n, we classified the pattern as "increasing"; if the frequency was < 80% that of the previous year, we classified the pattern as "decreasing"; if the frequency was between 80% and 120% of that of the previous year, we labeled the pattern as "stable".

The trend patterns enabled the retrieval of pairs of CEFs of the following four types of match patterns: (a) exact, i.e., all concatenated intervals have the same pattern; (b) opposite, i.e. all concatenated intervals have opposite patterns; (c) offset, i.e., the pattern matches with a lag of one or two years; and (d) approximate, i.e. a match for between 12 and 13 subintervals (i.e., a number smaller than 14 but not too off).

In addition, for quantitative CEFs such as A1c, creatinine, creatinine clearance, or body mass index, we plotted their value range distribution among all the cancer trials to visualize how patients of different value ranges for the selected eligibility features are included for cancer trials.

2.4   Trend Summarization

We further developed piecewise functions to summarize the usage trend of the CEFs between years 1999 and 2013 by multiple sub-functions, each applying to a certain time interval of the main function's domain (a subdomain). Our analysis included the following three steps. First, we calculated the usage of each CEF in each cancer type X in each year n, which ranges from 1999 to 2013. Second, to reduce the dimensions of the problem space, for each CEF, we partitioned the entire 15-year period into three 5-year intervals – 1999-2003, 2004-2008, and 2009-2013 – and calculated the average occurrences of the CEF for all cancer types within each sub-interval to get three values $X_{earliest}$, X_{middle}, X_{latest} using this formula:

$$X_c = \frac{1}{n}\sum_{i=1}^{n} fi$$

where subscript c is the earliest, middle, or latest time interval, n is the number of years in each interval (in this case n=5), i indicates each year in the time interval, and f_i is the occurrence of the CEF in the given year i for the given cancer type X. The possible relationships among these three measurements are illustrated in Fig. 1. Fig. 1(a) indicates $X_{earliest} < X_{middle} < X_{latest}$, while Fig. 1(b) indicates $X_{middle} < X_{earliest} < X_{latest}$. Finally, we named three temporal patterns: increasing, decreasing, and stable, which match Fig. 1 (a-c), Fig. 1(d-f), and Fig. 1 (g) respectively. We defined what accounts for larger than, smaller than, and equal to respectively by comparing the difference among $X_{earliest}$, X_{middle}, and X_{latest} to a delta selected programmatically.

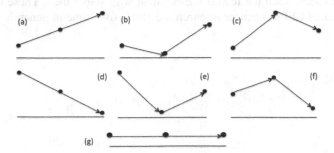

Fig. 1. The seven (a-g) possible relationships among $X_{earliest}$, X_{middle}, X_{latest}, where the x-axis represents time, while the y-axis represents the occurrence of a CEF across all cancer studies during the selected time period (earliest: 1999-2003, middle: 2004-2008, and latest: 2009-2013)

2.5   Network Analysis and Hierarchical Clustering

Using the information about the correlations among CEFs and similarities among cancers, we constructed the network of cancers and CEFs and calculated the network density and the centrality of each CEF (i.e., the count of cancers using this CEF at any time) or each center (i.e., the count of distinct CEFs used in trials of this cancer). We developed a 2-by-2 matrix of cancer type versus distinct CEF, in which the value of each cell was 0, -1, or 1, indicating that the CEF was classified as stable, decreasing, or increasing, respectively. Then, we hierarchically clustered cancer types by their similarity in (a) corresponding CEF centrality and (b) CEF trend patterns, respectively, using hierarchical clustering algorithm of MATLAB program. The pairwise distance between cancer types was measured using Jaccard Distance [22], which measures the percentage of nonzero elements that differ as follows:

$$J(C_i, C_j) = \frac{|C_i \cup C_j| - |C_i \cap C_j|}{|C_i \cup C_j|}$$

where C_i and C_j feature vectors of the cancer types, with i, j being 1, 2,.., 95, $i \neq j$. The smaller the Jaccard distance, the more similar were C_i and C_j.

3   Results

We identified 5,886 distinct CEFs that appeared in at least 20% of 99,109 cancer trials covering 95 cancer types. Their total occurrences in cancer trials were 54,927. The average number of CEFs used in a cancer research domain is 578.17. A total of 1,919 CEFs were used in research studies for only one cancer. We refer to these CEFs as cancer type-specific CEFs. On average, 78.72% of CEFs remain stable over time.

Fig. 2 plots the occurrences of CEFs of decreasing, increasing, or stable patterns in the 95 cancers. In all the cancers, most of the CEFs have stable usage patterns. Sixty-one cancers (64.2%) had more CEFs of increasing patterns than of decreasing patterns during the 15-year time period. Clinical trials for carcinoma of unknown primary site used the most CEFs, followed by skin and breast cancer, while trials for oropharyngeal cancer used the fewest CEFs, most with stable uses. These results imply that the uses of CEFs in cancer research are stable over time in general.

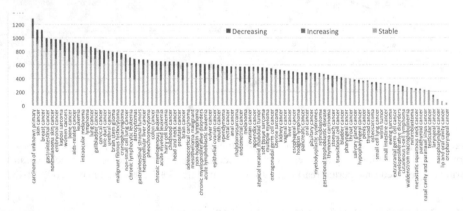

Fig. 2. Distributions of the CEF occurrences with decreasing or increasing patterns in the 95 cancer types: X-axis represents cancer type, Y-axis represents counts of CEFs in the trials for that cancer

The top 15 cancers ranked by the number of CEFs are *carcinoma of unknown primary origin, skin cancer, breast cancer, gastrointestinal cancer, nonmelanoma skin cancer, embryonal cancer, Kaposi's sarcoma, gynecologic cancers, bone cancer,*

AIDS-related cancer, leukemia, intraocular melanoma, lymphoma, lung cancer, and gallbladder cancer, where Kaposi's sarcoma and AIDS-related cancer are the same concept with different semantic representations.

The top 15 CEFs ranked by the number of cancers using them are *gender = both, minimum age = 18, platelets adverse event, transaminases, therapeutic brand of coal tar, Karnofsky performance status, serum creatinine level, SGOT - glutamate oxalo-acetate transaminase, alanine transaminase, allergy severity – severe, creatinine clearance, heart diseases, cardiac arrhythmia, operative surgical procedures,* and *pharmaceutical preparations.*

Fig. 3 displays the trends of three sample CEFs: (1) *hypersensitivity*; (2) *creatinine*; and (3) *creatinine clearance.* Since 2005, *hypersensitivity* has been adopted by clinical trials for up to 41% cancer types as a CEF, while previously its usage ranged between 5% and 10%. Meanwhile, starting in 2006, *creatinine clearance* has gradually replaced creatinine to indicate kidney function for the trials of between 18% and 27% of cancers.

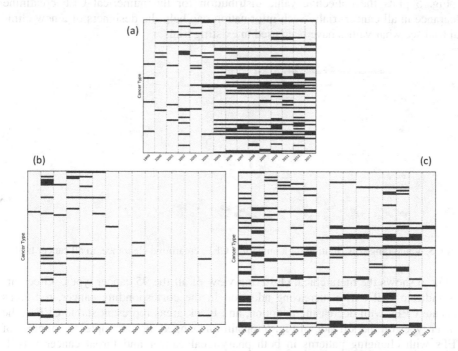

Fig. 3. Trends of (a) hypersensitivity, (b) creatinine, and (c) creatinine clearance in cancer trials. The y-axis indicates 95 cancer types and x-axis indicate years 1999-2013. Each blue bar indicates that CEF appears in at least 20% of the trials of the cancer type for the year.

Fig. 4 shows the similar trends of (a) *creatinine clearance* for female cancer and breast cancer research and (b) *serum creatinine level* for pancreatic cancer and brain cancer research, as well as the opposite trends between CEFs *pregnancy test negative* and *non-infiltrating lobular carcinoma* for skin cancer research.

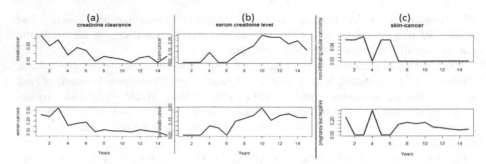

Fig. 4. (a) the similar trends of *creatinine clearance* between women cancer and breast cancer; (b) the similar trends of *serum creatinine level* between pancreatic cancer and brain cancer; (c) the opposite trends of *pregnancy-test negative* and *non-infiltrating nobular carcinoma* in skin cancer research

Fig. 5 plots the collective value distribution for the numerical CEF creatinine clearance in all cancer trials. Such information can help the designers of a new clinical trial see what values have been used in existing trials.

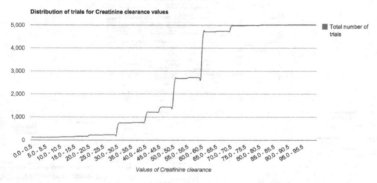

Fig. 5. Value range distribution for a numerical CEF, creatinine clearance, in all cancer trials

Fig. 6 shows the hierarchical clustering view of all the 95 cancer types. Green areas indicate CEFs with increasing adoption in the corresponding cancer, red areas indicate CEFs with decreasing adoption, and black areas represent stable CEFs. The cancer types on the left side of Fig. 6 remain unchanged. For example, the number of CEFs with changing patterns in both pharyngeal cancer and throat cancer was 1, where the former was the subtype of the latter. The Jaccard distance between these two cancer types was 0, which means that the classification results of the CEFs used in these cancer types are the same. The total numbers of classified CEFs in the skin and breast cancers were 210 and 250, respectively. The Jaccard distance between these two cancer types was 0.46, which means that they share 54% of the CEFs that have the same trends in both cancers.

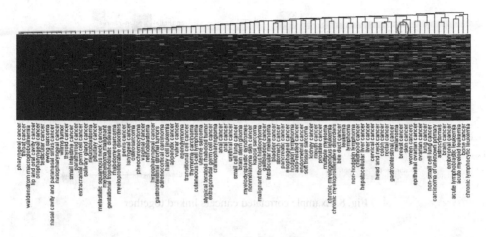

Fig. 6. The hierarchical clustering view of all 95 cancer types clustered by their similar CEF trends (*: the red circle highlights breast and skin cancers)

As shown in Fig. 7, five clusters within which cancer types with similar centrality were grouped. Green areas indicate CEFs with increasing adoption in the corresponding cancer, red shows CEFs with decreasing adoption, and black represents stable CEFs. The leftmost cluster (linked by red lines on the top) includes breast cancer, skin cancer, women cancer, cervical cancer, head and neck cancer, colon cancer, and rectal cancer, gastrointestinal cancer, lung cancer, and non-small cell lung cancer.

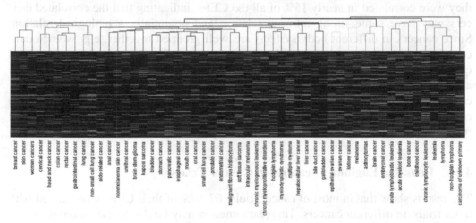

Fig. 7. The hierarchical clustering view of the cancer types that had at least 99 CEFs grouped by their similar centrality, i.e., count of CEFs connected to each cancer

We took the top 30 scored cancer-pairs and built a network based on their connections, as shown in Fig. 8. Each cancer-pair's score was assigned by calculating the prevalence of the pairwise-relatedness of each two cancers among all CEFs. It can be seen that biologically related cancers are clustered into same group. The group for women cancers, for circulatory system related cancers, and for alimentary system-related cancers were all closely clustered. The similarity between skin cancer and breast cancer was previously reported [23].

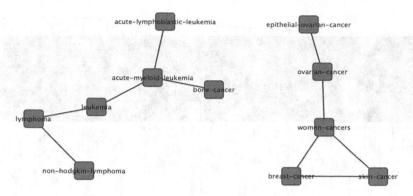

Fig. 8. Example correlated cancers linked together

4   Discussion

4.1   Literature-Based Results Evaluation

Our network analysis shows that some CEFs are important for a specific cancer, e.g. "communicable diseases" is a cluster center for acute lymphoblastic leukemia. Prior research has shown that infection plays a very important role in children acute lymphoblastic leukemia [24]. Although we used a rigorous definition of correlation, the top 30 cancer pairs' scores were very high—over 50 out of 378 CEFs, which means they were correlated in nearly 15% of all the CEFs, indicating that the correlated cancers may have some strong intrinsic relation and potentially a biological relation. Since cancers in different body systems are well grouped together, e.g. women cancer, group for circulatory system related cancer, group for alimentary system-related cancers, future studies are warranted to test the existence of biological relations among these identified correlated cancers. For example, astrocytoma is a neurologic cancer inside brain; our results showed this connection. Prior research studies have confirmed the relation between breast cancer and skin cancer. In general, some of the results confirmed both biological knowledge and existing research findings.

4.2   Reusable Eligibility Features in Cancer Trials

The results show that in most of cancer trials, 67.40% of their CEFs were shared with other trials on different cancers. This phenomenon may be due to the common procedure of clinical trials or the similar conditions for all cancers. The cancer type-specific CEFs contain special information while common CEFs reveal the similarity in eligibility feature selection among different cancer trials. The cancer-specific CEFs tend to be distributed unevenly across all cancers, which may be associated with several possible explanations. It may be due to the measurability for a certain disease or the level of communication by the researchers in this domain or even the popularity of the disease research. Those factors may cause the high variation of cancer-specific CEFs. As a result, one can argue that those CEFs may contain less useful information. However, when we develop the cancer research knowledge network using the CEFs, the cancer-specific CEFs could contain information that could be useful in differentiating research among different types of cancers. For common CEFs, they are more robust and sometimes are reflections of the common procedures of the cancer domain.

4.3   Implications for Clinical Research Standards Development

The field of biomedical informatics, including the subfield of clinical research informatics, is becoming burdened by the proliferation of clinical research information standards, available or under development, and their consequent sparse adoption by clinical researchers and vendors. To supplement the current top-down model of "standards development by experts followed by dissemination to users", we propose a temporal knowledge acquisition method for uncovering frequently used data elements in clinical research text to facilitate community-based knowledge sharing and empirically founded standards development. We hypothesize that this method can identify content frequently used by the research community and thereby increase the adoption of standards derived "from researchers and for researchers".

4.4   Limitations and Future Work

This study has several limitations that we hope will motivate future work. First, in this study, we focused on discrete, UMLS-recognizable common eligibility features, such as A1c, creatinine clearance, and serum creatinine level. We based this decision on the limitation in our current text-mining technique that can only extract n-grams without syntactic processing at the sentence level. We did not extract contextual clinical outcome variables, such as "*heart attack after stroke within the past 5 years*", whose reuse patterns may be more useful to clinical trial investigators. One of our future directions is to enhance our tag mining method to capture such long phrases and analyze their trends and cancer trials with similar patterns for such long phrases.

Second, persistent data quality deficiencies in the ClinicalTrials.gov remain a barrier to such studies. We observed dependencies among cancer names used in ClinicalTrials.gov, such as "women cancers", "breast cancer", and "ovarian cancer"; the former is a more general concept to the latter two. Such dependencies can interfere with aggregation studies across cancers. More work is needed to improve the indexing of clinical trials by precise medical condition terminologies on ClinicalTrials.gov.

Moreover, the eligibility criteria for clinical trials almost always expressed as separate inclusion and exclusion criteria. In this study, we combined them together for several reasons. First, they all contain certain level of information indicating the conditions of interest. Second, there is no standard for how researchers should state the eligibility section for ClinicalTrials.gov. Thus, it is hard to clearly separate the inclusion from exclusion criteria.

Our lab has recently developed a database called COMPACT (Commonalities in Target Populations of Clinical Trials) using the text-mining results from ClinicalTrials.gov. We downloaded all the XML-format trial files from ClinicalTrials.gov. We made all the structured characteristics of trials readily computable by extracting them from trials and storing them in a relational database. Using

COMPACT, we can refine the trend and network analysis of CEFs by specifying various characteristics of trials, such as phase, study type (interventional/ observational), and intervention type (i.e., drug, device, and procedure). For example, we can analyze the trend of CEFs of phases-3 medication intervention trials involving female patients 75 years old or older with COMPACT. This resource can potentially make the analyses reported in this paper more fine-grained and more readily available for medical conditions other than cancer. In the future, we will perform such analyses with the hope of discovering granular patterns in the eligibility criteria designs for various diseases.

5   Conclusions

We contributed an analytical method to identify the most common eligibility criteria of cancer clinical trials and to identify those criteria with increasing or decreasing adoption patterns in different cancer studies over time. This method can potentially generalize to other disease domains. Our data-driven approach to acquiring clinical research knowledge from text has the potential to supplement existing expert-based methods for clinical research standards development and hence may increase the likelihood of the adoption of those standards.

Acknowledgments. This study was funded by the National Library of Medicine grant R01 LM009886.

References

1. Kamal, J., Pasuparthi, K., Rogers, P., Buskirk, J., Mekhjian, H.S.: Using and Information Warehouse to Screen Patients for Clinical Trials: A Prototype. In: American Medical Informatics Association Annual Symposium, Washington, DC, p. 1004 (2005)
2. Nammuni, K., Pickering, C., Modgil, S., Montgomery, A., Hammond, P., Wyatt, J.C., et al.: Design-a-trial: a rule-based decision support system for clinical trial design. Knowledge-Based Systems 17, 121–129 (2004)
3. Musen, M.A., Tu, S.W., Das, A.K., Shahar, Y.: EON: a component-based approach to automation of protocol-directed therapy. JAMIA 3, 367–388 (1996)
4. Musen, M.A., Rohn, J.A., Fagan, L.M., Shortliffe, E.H.: Knowledge engineering for a clinical trial advice system: uncovering errors in protocol specification. Bulletin du Cancer 74, 291–296 (1987)
5. Shortliffe, E.H., Scott, A.C., Bischoff, M.B., Campbell, A.B., Melle, W.V., Jacobs, C.D.: ONCOCIN: An expert system for oncology protocol management. In: Seventh International Joint Conference on Artificial Intelligence, Vancouver, BC (1981)
6. Weng, C., Tu, S.W., Sim, I., Richesson, R.: Formal representation of eligibility criteria: a literature review. J. Biomed. Inform. 43, 451–467 (2010)
7. Milian, K., Bucur, A., van Harmelen, F.: Building a Library of Eligibility Criteria to Support Design of Clinical Trials. In: ten Teije, A., Völker, J., Handschuh, S., Stuckenschmidt, H., d'Acquin, M., Nikolov, A., Aussenac-Gilles, N., Hernandez, N. (eds.) EKAW 2012. LNCS (LNAI), vol. 7603, pp. 327–336. Springer, Heidelberg (2012)

8. Luo, Z., Miotto, R., Weng, C.: A human-computer collaborative approach to identifying common data elements in clinical trial eligibility criteria. Journal of Biomedical Informatics 46, 33–39 (2013)
9. Niland, J., Dorr, D., El Saadawi, G., Embi, P., Richesson, R.L., Sim, I., et al.: Knowledge Representation of Eligibility Criteria in Clinical Trials. In: American Medical Informatics Association Annual Symposium, Chicago (2007)
10. Gennari, J., Sklar, D., Silva, J.: Cross-tool communication: From protocol authoring to eligibility determination. In: Proc. AMIA Symp., pp. 199–203 (2001)
11. Weng, C., Gennari, J.H., Fridsma, D.B.: User-centered semantic harmonization: a case study. J. Biomed. Inform. 40, 353–364 (2007)
12. Weng, C., Fridsma, D.B.: A call for collaborative semantics harmonization. In: AMIA Annu. Symp. Proc., p. 1142 (2006)
13. Tenenbaum, J.D., Sansone, S.-A., Haendel, M.: A sea of standards for omics data: sink or swim? Journal of the American Medical Informatics Association: JAMIA 21, 200–203 (2014)
14. Bhattacharya, S., Cantor, M.N.: Analysis of eligibility criteria representation in industry-standard clinical trial protocols. J. Biomed. Inform. 46, 805–813 (2013)
15. Hao, T., Rusanov, A., Boland, M.R., Weng, C.: Clustering clinical trials with similar eligibility criteria features. J. Biomed. Inform. (February 1, 2014)
16. Boland, M.R., Miotto, R., Weng, C.: A method for probing disease relatedness using common clinical eligibility criteria. Studies in Health Technology and Informatics 192, 481–485 (2013)
17. McCray, A.T.: Better access to information about clinical trials. Ann. Intern. Med. 133, 609–614 (2000)
18. Miotto, R., Weng, C.: Unsupervised mining of frequent tags for clinical eligibility text indexing. Journal of Biomedical Informatics 46, 1145–1151 (2013)
19. Lindberg, D.A., Humphreys, B.L., McCray, A.T.: The Unified Medical Language System. Methods Inf. Med. 32, 281–291 (1993)
20. Luo, Z., Johnson, S.B., Weng, C.: Semi-Automatically Inducing Semantic Classes of Clinical Research Eligibility Criteria Using UMLS and Hierarchical Clustering. In: AMIA Annu. Symp. Proc., vol. 2010, pp. 487–491 (2010)
21. Fisher, R.A.: On the probable error of a coefficient of correlation deduced from a small sample. Metron 1, 3–32 (1921)
22. Jaccard, P.: Lois de distribution florale. Bulletin de la Socíeté Vaudoise des Sciences Naturelles 38, 67–130 (1902)
23. Ho, W.L., Comber, H., Hill, A.D., Murphy, G.M.: Malignant melanoma and breast carcinoma: a bidirectional correlation. Ir. J. Med. Sci. 180, 901–903 (2011)
24. Hishamuddin, P.: The association between acute lymphoblastic leukemia in children and Helicobacter pylori as the marker for sanitation. BMC Res. Notes 5, 345 (2012)

A Conceptual Framework of Information Analysis and Modelling for E-health

William W. Song

Informatics, Dalarna University, Sweden
wso@du.se

Abstract. E-health (or e-healthcare) aims at applying modern information and telecommunication technologies in the healthcare sector. Recently, more and more research attention has been paid to this area, from clinic data analysis to patient record management. If we say the e-health has been mainly dealing with patient data analysis and various disease diagnosis at its early time, nowadays various data sources, such as social network, physician and patients' blogs, and various monitoring data (like sensors attached to PD patients at home) are widely used for aid of better disease diagnosis through gathering richer experts' knowledge and expertise, richer data (from patients, diseases, diagnosis, medical experiments, etc.) for analysis, and quicker (or better timely) access to various resources (e.g. telemedicine) pervasively.

Keywords: e-health, healthcare informatics, tele-medication, e-patient records, remote sensor motoring.

1 Introduction

E-health (or e-healthcare), aims at applying modern information and telecommunication technologies (ICT) in the healthcare sector, is becoming a hot research topic due to its wide involvement in not only clinic care for patients, but governmental healthcare policy making and public concerns, e.g. blog medical consultation, as well. According to WHO, e-Health is defined as: "… the use of information and communication technologies (ICT) for health to, for example, treat patients, pursue research, educate students, track diseases and monitor public health" [1]. The term e-health was thought for the first time to be proposed in 1999 when Mitchell, at the telemedicine conference in London pointed out that "e-health can be considered to be the health industry's equivalent of e-commerce," and this could be one key for understanding the sense of e-health: just medical informatics and telematics on the shop shelves, a fashionable name for something already existing but otherwise difficult to sell [2]. Since then, more and more research attention has been paid to this area, from clinic data analysis to patient record management. If we say the e-health has been mainly dealing with patient data analysis and various disease diagnosis at its early time, nowadays various data sources, such as social network, physician and patients' blogs, and various monitoring data (like sensors attached to PD patients at home) are widely used for

X. Zheng et al. (Eds.): ICSH 2014, LNCS 8549, pp. 142–147, 2014.

aid of better disease diagnosis through gathering richer experts' knowledge and expertise, richer data (from patients, diseases, diagnosis, medical experiments, etc.) for analysis, and quicker (or better timely) access to various resources (e.g. telemedicine) pervasively.

Usually, e-health involves these aspects related to healthcare activities using information systems (informatics).

- Electronic health records – mainly focusing on communication of patient data between healthcare professionals.
- E-Prescription – an electronic transmission of prescriptions between doctors and pharmacists, as well as patients.
- Telemedicine – remote physical treatments, including distance-monitoring of patients functions.
- Healthcare information systems – considering management of healthcare data, including demographic data, lab data, and biologic data (e.g. bio-ontology).

In this position paper, we attempt to provide an overview of current e-healthcare research and development with some case studies conducted at our research group. We will propose a conceptual model for e-healthcare data and information, followed by a discussion of research trends in the area and finally brief our case studies in Parkinson Disease monitoring methods and clinic registration systems for local communities in Sweden.

2   A General Conceptual Model for E-healthcare Data

Nowadays, there is a huge amount of data used for healthcare directly or indirectly. It is necessary to suggest a conceptual model for the healthcare data/information in order to gain an overview of them and a good insight of its complexity – various diverse information sources, complex structures, and intertwisted connections and relations. We consider a three-layered data model, in which the foundational layered data are of two sorts: core data – directly coming from patients, diseases, and diagnoses (physicists records), and peripheral data - governmental policies, insurance information, social network data, medical professionals' blogs, medical website data, etc.

For the first sort, usually there are three categories: 1) The patient data include clinic visit data, individual treatment records, histories, and family data; 2) The disease data contains normal disease ontology, typical symptoms information, and bio-evolution data; and 3) information about treatment processes, diagnosis procedures, medication data and effects.

The second sort of data fall in these categories: 1) managerial data such as governmental healthcare policies and decisions, healthcare insurance information and regulations, organizational health benefits, etc.; 2) healthcare public information sources such as health websites, professionals' blogs, television special channels for healthcare, and public sciences of medicines and medication knowledge; and 3) experimental data, both for experts and public, including medications, biological lab data, etc.

The intermediate layer of the healthcare information consists of a great number of information systems maintaining these data mentioned above. It is typical that at moment each hospital, even a community healthcare centre, uses an information system (or a clinic database system) to store, sort, retrieve, and manage patient information, such as registration accounts, clinic visit information, treatment records, remission documents, and so on.

There are three key functions provided at this layer: 1) information management (including knowledge management), i.e. gathering and maintaining healthcare data, validating and verifying them for integrity, and reasoning and correcting them for precision and correctness; 2) information sharing and integration, e.g. patients' registration information can be shared among a few local clinics, e.g. children's vaccination records could be shared among different regions or even countries, and e.g. people's registration data, when they registered at different places or authorities, could be integrated and stored in a central database system; 3) information dissemination, aiming at making the healthcare information available to patients, experts, and public (note that we need to distinguish the information available for   private to that for public).

The outer layer is an extension to information dissemination. Here we focus on the information and communication technologies applied to the healthcare information, so that people can access to them, query them, and interact with medical experts and other people. There are three fields seeming to be promising in the future. The first is self-checking, self-testing, and self-diagnosis. With more and more healthcare information and knowledge become available to public, people are more capable to examine their own health situations, watching their nutrition, monitoring their medical treatment, and keeping adequate physical exercises. In other words, people pay more attention to their health and are able to do so.

The second is remote monitoring. This issue is closely related to the above one. Nowadays, with a wide application of "wireless sensor network (WSN)" systems, patients could be monitored pervasively, i.e. where they are, be they at home, at work, or even travelling abroad. A knowledge based Information Systems for WSN (KIS4WSN) [10] is able to timely record and store your physical conditions and report to the healthcare monitoring centre. A recent publication at Science Magazine [8] even discussed how to use sensor network nodes attached to a body in order to monitor various micro-messages our body emits. "When mounted on the skin, modern sensors, circuits, radios, and power supply systems have the potential to provide clinical-quality health monitoring capabilities for continuous use, beyond the confines of traditional hospital or laboratory facilities."

The third one is to apply powerful data analytics for healthcare management and disease diagnosis. We are at the age of big data, of which a large amount is from medical and healthcare or related domains. As pointed out by W. Raghupathi and V. Raghupathi [6], "Big data in healthcare refers to electronic health data sets so large and complex that they are difficult (or impossible) to manage with traditional software and/or hardware; nor can they be easily managed with traditional or common data management tools and methods [3]". Similarly, in the field of monitoring human's skin conditions, "the most well-developed component technologies are, however, broadly available only in hard, planar formats. As a result, existing options in system design are unable to effectively accommodate integration with the soft, textured, curvilinear, and time-dynamic surfaces of the skin." [8] For example, it has been very easy for a patient to consult experts (or others) though she could only go to few local hospitals to see doctors in face. With different information channels such as through clinic consultations, experts' advices, even friends' recommendations, and others' suggestion, becoming available, one could get more information and knowledge about the problems and find a right or suitable solution.

3   Some Examples

3.1   PD Monitoring

One investigation we have pursued is to collect, sort, and analyze symptom data for PD patients via various sources, including images, voices, motions, as well as daily activities [5]. We adopt the methods of pattern recognition and quantitative analysis for these cases and develop diagnosis systems. PD is a progressive neurological movement disorder associated with a variety of motor and non-motor symptoms. In a clinical setting today, the state of the art is to use clinical rating scales such as the Unified Parkinson's Disease Rating Scale (UPDRS) and the 39-item PD Question-naire (PDQ-39). Problem is the use of these scales in clinical practice is accompanied with a number of limitations including large within- and between-clinician variability in ratings, low resolution assessments, the need for a clinician's presence, among others. Thus, telemedicine-based systems, coupled with statistical and machine learning methods, can be useful for deriving quantitative, objective (clinician-independent), unobtrusive and valid outcome measures which can improve the clinical management of PD by providing solutions to deliver healthcare by remote monitoring of patients [7]. We have developed a telemedicine framework for remote collection, processing and presentation of symptom data of advanced PD patients.

3.2   Registration Information Systems

Integration of registration documents has long been a problem to make various healthcare data, stored in different medical and clinic information systems in different locations, available to public, especially to patients when seeking clinic visits. A major reason is that most of the documents are maintained at low quality, such as incomplete information, lack of necessary links among the related documents due to multi-registrations, and heterogeneous structures of storing data. The National Quality Registers (NKRs) [4] is a system of quality tools used in Sweden, for continuous improvement and provision of a good healthcare. It contains individual data concerning patient problems, medical interventions, and post-treatment outcomes, aiming at encompassing all healthcare production. There is a trend emerging among the healthcare administration and managements, that the register results should be made available to the public over the Internet so that the citizens can have direct access to their own care units as well as the other care units (hospitals and clinics), providing a selection freedom to the citizens to choose a care unit, which is convenient and trustable, and has good quality [4].

4   Conclusion

E-healthcare is becoming an increasingly strong research subject due to massive public interests in various aspects of biologic knowledge, nutrition information, human bodies, genetic researches, healthy rearing, medical treatment processes, very much like people's enthusiasm in modern physics, planet science, and particle physics. One reason is that at the Web time, it is extremely convenient for people to access different resources for what they want, particularly things concerning health problems.

Of course, overwhelmingly large amount of healthcare and medical-related information is indeed a problem ("big data" problem) while we benefit from that. A practical set of data analysis approaches have to established, which can compare data, find patterns, and explore them further. Simply processing methods for complex data are certainly not a good practice – neither a timely solution to identify, say critical diseases, nor a necessary one to get too much information for it. We believe to gain semantics from "vast data" – conceptualization – is the only way out. We can categorize massive information, in a way that makes sense to us and anticipate discoveries by following visual cues and nudges, allowing the data to intuitively guide us to the answers we seek and predict future outcomes based on insights. All this forms an information (knowledge) analysis hierarchical structure of methods with four levels: statistic methods, conceptual modelling methods, semantic extraction methods, and knowledge support system methods.

Based on this hierarchical structure, we will build up a virtual organization for e-health (VO-e-health) which is able to provide these functions: synthetic information analysis for medical diagnosis (healthcare), healthcare information management, and pervasive patients' activity monitoring.

References

1. eHealth: the Future Direction of Clinical Care, in Embedding Informatics in Clinic Education, http://www.eiceresources.org/learning-to-manage-health-information/preparing-clinicians-for-the-future-ehealth-and-the-clinical-curriculum
2. Mea, V.D.: What is e-Health (2): The death of telemedicine (2001), http://www.jmir.org/2001/2/e22/
3. Frost & Sullivan: Drowning in Big Data? Reducing information technology complexities and costs for healthcare organizations, http://www.emc.com/collateral/analyst-reports/frost-sullivan-reducing-information-technology-complexities-ar.pdf
4. Halilovic, A.: What is national quality registries? report, Dalarna Lansting, Sweden (2014)
5. Khan, T., Memedi, M., Song, W., Westin, J.: A mobile-based telemedicine framework for automated Parkinson's disease symptom assessment, Beijing, China (July 2014) (accepted by ICSH 2014)

6. Raghupathi, W., Raghupathi, V.: Big Data analytics in healthcare: promise and potential, Health Information Science and Systems. BioMed. Central (the Open Access Publisher) 2, 3 (2014)
7. Westin, J., Dougherty, M., Nyholm, D., Groth, T.: A home environment test battery for status assessment in patients with advanced Parkinson's disease. Computer Methods and Programs in Biomedicine 98(1), 27–35 (2010)
8. Xu, S., et al.: Soft Microfluidic Assemblies of Sensors, Circuits, and Radios for the Skin. Science 344(6179), 70–74 (2014), doi:10.1126/science.1250169
9. Why Natural Analytics Matters, report, at Qlik.com
10. Zhang, S., Liu, X., Song, W.: Using Knowledge-based Information Systems to Support Management of Wireless Sensor Networking System, Croatia (October 2014) (submitted to ISD 2014)

Extended Abstract: Combining Statistical Analysis and Markov Models with Public Health Data to Infer Age-Specific Background Mortality Rates for Hepatitis C Infection in the U.S.

Shan Liu[1], Lauren E. Cipriano[2], and Jeremy D. Goldhaber-Fiebert[3]

[1] University of Washington, Seattle, Washington, USA
[2] Ivey Business School, London, Ontario, Canada
[3] Stanford University, Stanford, California, USA

Abstract. Chronic hepatitis C (HCV) is a significant public health problem affecting 2.7-3.9 million Americans. Quantifying mortality rates of HCV-infected individuals permits more accurate estimates of the potential benefits of HCV screening and treatment. With 5% of older Americans infected with HCV, cost-effectiveness analyses of expanded HCV screening and treatment require methods to appropriately quantify differential mortality risks. No single study contains data needed to estimate subgroup-specific prevalence of HCV, risk factor status, and mortality risks. We developed a combined modeling approach to infer risk-group-specific mortality rates for chronically HCV-infected U.S. adults. We incorporated estimates from public health data into a Markov model to infer the age-, sex-, race-, risk-, and HCV infection status-specific mortality rates that best fit the overall age-specific population mortality rates.

1 Statistical Analyses on HCV Prevalence and Risk Factors

We estimated the prevalence of risk factors and the prevalence of HCV among high- and low-risk individuals stratified by age, sex and race using data from the U.S. National Health and Nutrition Examination Survey (NHANES) (2001-2008). We defined a high-risk person as someone having a history of injection drug use, transfusion prior to 1992, or greater than 20 lifetime sex partners. We combined all survey years to estimate prevalence for the 1952-1961 birth cohort in the base case, using the 1962-1971 birth cohort prevalence in sensitivity analyses (n = 5,654). We used logistic regression to predict the prevalence of being high-risk based on sex, race, and age accounting for sample weighting and NHANES complex sampling design. Similarly, we used logistic regression to predict the prevalence of individuals with HCV antibodies using sex, race, risk status, and age. We estimated HCV antibody prevalence for subgroups above age 40. Depending on subgroup, 15-31% are high-risk, and HCV antibody prevalence is higher for high-risk individuals (11-17%) compared to low-risk individuals (2-3%).

X. Zheng et al. (Eds.): ICSH 2014, LNCS 8549, pp. 148–149, 2014.
© Springer International Publishing Switzerland 2014

2   Statistical Analyses on Background Mortality

We developed a combined modeling approach to infer necessary risk-group-specific mortality rates for chronically HCV-infected U.S. adults. We analyzed the NHANES III–linked mortality data in which HCV status was assessed from 1988 to 1994 with mortality follow-up of the same persons through 2006 (n = 15,892). We constructed Cox proportional hazard models to estimate the mortality hazard ratios for all-cause death by sex, race, HCV, risk status, interaction between HCV and risk status, age, and age-squared variables for people between ages 17-60, excluding cases with missing risk information. Controlling for age, we used four hazard ratios (male, black, HCV positive, and high risk) to calculate the 16 mortality hazard ratios. Result showed all-cause mortality rates are higher in men (HR: 1.3 [1.1-1.7]); blacks (HR: 1.7 [1.5-2.1]); high-risk individuals (HR: 1.4 [1.0-1.9]); and HCV infected individuals (HR: 3.5 [2.0-6.0]). To adjust for non-liver related death, we adjusted the ratio for HCV infection down using a factor of 0.8 since it is estimated that for HCV-infected individuals, 20% of mortality is liver-related.

Using the 16 estimated hazard ratios, we calculated the population-weighted average mortality to match the 2006 U.S. life-table over age 50-100, based on the prevalence of HCV and risk status by sex and race from NHANES (2001-2008) data analyses and the U.S. 2009 census distribution for people aged 50-54 (non-black male 44%, non-black female 45%, black male 5%, and black female 6%). To avoid overestimation of death in the older ages, we linearly attenuated the 16 hazard ratios starting from age 70 down to 1.0 by age 100. We inferred sixteen life tables by sex, race, risk, and HCV infection status. Result showed that within each subgroup, the life expectancy of high-risk individuals is up to 3 years shorter; similarly, the life expectancy of chronically HCV-infected individuals is up to 9 years shorter.

Apply Autocorrelation and Forward Difference to Measure Vital Signs Using Ordinary Camera

Letian Sun[1], Li Liu[1,2], Ye Wei[1], Jun Zhong[1], Dashi Luo[1],
Ming Liu[3], and Hamed Monkaresi[4]

[1] School of Information Science and Engineering, Lanzhou University, Gansu, China
{sunyt_13,liliu,weiy13,zhongj13,luodsh12}@lzu.edu.cn
[2] School of Computing, National University of Singapore, Singapore
[3] Faculty of Computer and Information Science, Southwest University,
Chongqing, China
liuming9902@gmail.com
[4] School of Electrical and Information Engineering, The University of Sydney,
Sydney, Australia
monkaresi@gmail.com

Abstract. Measuring heart rate by portable equipments becomes more and more popular. Current methods such as wavelet, fast fourier transform, peak detection, have been used to analyze heart rate. However, in some cases these methods are ineffective. For example, as a denoising tool, wavelet is not necessary in a few cases. One of the main challenges is determining an effective size of sliding window for heart rate detection when using peak detection. In addition, the time complexity of fast fourier transform is large which can increase the processing time that is not desirable for real-time heart rate detection systems. In this paper, we introduce autocorrelation and forward difference to count heart rate based on the features of cardiac cycle. The results show that our method is good enough so that it can be applied to non-invasive health state detection. And the time complexity of our method is satisfactory.

Keywords: vital sign, heart rate, autocorrelation, forward difference.

1 Introduction

In order to assess the basic body functions and obtain health condition, vital signs, such as body temperature, heart rate (HR), blood pressure (BP) and respiratory rate (RR), are important indicators. At present, health-related portable devices which can measure vital signs become popular. For example, Fitbit Inc. [1], which is devoted to helping people to be healthier, is famous for its devices that can measure walking steps, sleep quality and other health-related metrics. Besides, some practical health-related mobile applications are developed. Moves [2], a free mobile app can be used as a step counter and a calorie counter. And it can measure the distance and duration of walk or run. Instant Heart Rate [3], which is an Android app developed by Azumio Inc., is used for

X. Zheng et al. (Eds.): ICSH 2014, LNCS 8549, pp. 150–159, 2014.

measuring HR. In addition, some devices that need to cooperate with mobile phone are manufactured. AliveCor Heart Monitor [4], which is a combination of smart phone application and electrodes, can record, display, store, and transfer single-channel electrocardiogram (ECG). With the popularity of laptop and smart phone which have more and more strong processing capacity, people can understand their own health condition quickly, easily and cheaply.

In real life, the changes of many vital signs are cyclical, such as HR, RR, ECG changes. HR, as one kind of vital sign, is usually described as the number of heart beats per minute (BPM). The periodic beats of heart can cause periodic change of the volume of vessel. Then some features, such as temperature and light, change. Besides, bioelectricity changes cyclically as well . There are some non-intrusive methods to get HR. The cardiac cycle causes changes in temperature, especially at carotid vessel. Then a wavelet-based measurement is brought forward in paper [5]. Chekmenev et al. used remote passive thermal imaging to acquire the data which reflects the change of heat [5]. In order to obtain the HR, Pursche et al. used independent component analysis (ICA) , peak detection and the fast Fourier transform (FFT) to process the data extracted from the video of a participant's face [6]. By applying ICA on the color channels in video recordings, Poh et al. extracted the blood volume pulse from the facial regions, and then obtained HR and RR [7].

Because vital signs change with time and feature value can be extracted at every time point, time series is introduced in our study. A time series is a sequence of data points, and the points are measured in time spaced at uniform time intervals [8]. Therefore, the sequence which shows the change of temperature or light can be regard as a time series. The similarity of two time series (STTS) which have the same size is used to describe the degree of correlation of the two series. When every pair of data points from two time series at the same time point has equal value and the same trend, the value of STTS is maximal. The more different the value and trend are, the smaller the value of STTS is. Generally, the value range of STTS is [-1,1].

In another study [5], the continuous wavelet transform (CWT) and inverse continuous wavelet transform (ICWT) are used to denoise the time series. HR and RR are computed by counting the maxima. We find each periodic change can be identified obviously in some time series exhibited in paper [5], so denoising algorithm is unnecessary in some cases. From another perspective, as a peak detection tool, wavelet analysis greatly facilitates the compute of the following compute of HR and RR. A simple algorithm to compute HR is to count only maxima or only minima. If the value of a data point in a sliding window which have specified size is maximum or minimum, then this point represents one heart beat . However, the size of sliding window is difficult to determine. The noise can make it more difficult. In [6], FFT is introduced to obtain HR. For a time series which contains n data points, FFT take $O(n \log n)$ time. Though FFT can achieve an accurate estimate, its time complexity is a bit large.

In this paper, we introduce a new approach with low time complexity called FDAC for HR detection. This approach is based on forward difference (FD) and autocorrelation (AC). AC can be used to calculate the STTS while FD can make the raw data fluctuate around a stable value.

2   Methods

2.1   Experimental Set-Up

In our experiment, we record the continuous change of light by placing a camera around fingertip in a well-lit environment, the subject should keep still in the meantime. Fig. 1 shows how to record the change. The camera is the rear camera of HUAWEI G700-U00 and have 8 megapixels. The recording color mode is set to RGB. The resolution of the camera is set to 640*480, and the video is recorded with a length of 1 minute at 30 frames per second (fps). Each frame extracted from the video is converted to grayscale, and the average value of all pixels of each grayscale is considered as its feature value. The feature values form a time series.

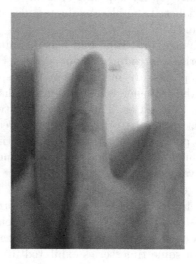

Fig. 1. How to record the continuous change of light

Fig. 2 shows an example that feature values change with increasing serial number of frame.

2.2   Analysis of the Time Series

Because of the regularity of feature values, we introduce AC to process the time series showed in Fig. 2. For time series, the AC represents the correlation between values at different times.

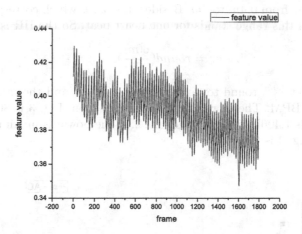

Fig. 2. An example that feature values change with increasing serial number of frame. The x-axis represents the serial number of each frame and it start with 1. The y-axis represents corresponding feature value.

Let $X = x_1, x_2, \ldots, x_{n-1}, x_n$ be a time series. Data points $x_1, x_2, \ldots, x_{n-1}, x_n$ are spaced at equal time intervals.

In [8], Box et al. mention that for a discrete time series, the most satisfactory estimate of AC at kth lag is

$$r_k = \frac{c_k}{c_0} \tag{1}$$

in which

$$c_k = \frac{1}{n} \sum_{t=1}^{n-k} (x_t - \overline{x})(x_{t+k} - \overline{x}) \tag{2}$$

In formula (2), n is the amount of the data points, $\overline{x}$ is the mean value of X.

Let $X1 = x_t, x_{t+1}, \ldots, x_{n-k-1}, x_{n-k}$, and $X2 = x_{t+k}, x_{t+k+1}, \ldots, x_{n-1}, x_n$. The more the STTS between $X1$ and $X2$ is, the more the AC of $X1$ and $X2$ is. The value range of r_k is $[-1, 1]$, and the correlation between $X1$ and $X2$ will be stronger as the absolute value r_k becomes greater.

Here we treat the serial number of frame as time point, then the AC based on the specified lag k is computed. Fig. 3 shows the AC result based on the series in Fig. 2, in which the x-axis represents the lag and it starts with 0, ends with 60. The y-axis represents corresponding AC. Besides, to compare with AC, FFT is used to analyse the data in Fig. 2. Fig. 4 shows FFT result.

As showed in Fig. 3, when lag is 0, the AC is 1, and when the lag is 21, the AC is a maximal value. In fact, 21 can be regarded as the amount of frames occupied by one heart beat. Generally speaking, the frequency of heart ranges from 0.4Hz to 2.0Hz. Therefore, if the sampling rate is mHz, the frames a heart beat occupy range from $0.4m$ to $2m$. Besides, the lag k which corresponding the maximal value in this range stands for one heart beat. So the HR is:

$$hr = round(\frac{60m}{k}), \qquad (3)$$

function $round$ let $\frac{60m}{k}$ round towards nearest integer , and the metrics of calculated result is BPM. Therefore, the HR obtained from Fig. 3 is 86. In Fig. 4, when frequency is 1.406Hz in the range $[0.4, 2.0]$, the power is maximal. The HR obtained from Fig. 4 is 84.

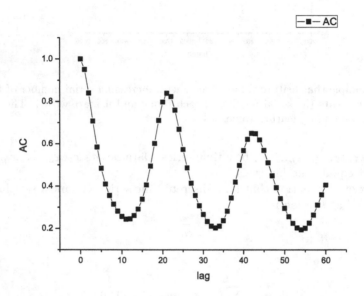

Fig. 3. The AC result of data in Fig. 2

In the actual test, subject cannot stay still ideally. Although the time series shows high regularity on the time dimension, the raw data do not fluctuate around a stable value. This make the regularity on the vision a little pale. FD is introduced to process raw data showed in Fig. 2. FD is a finite difference, and in our time series $\triangle x_i$ is defined as:

$$\triangle x_i = x_{i+1} - x_i \qquad (4)$$

Then we can get time series $\triangle X = \triangle x_1, \triangle x_2, \dots, \triangle x_{n-2}, \triangle x_{n-1}$. Fig. 5 shows the difference result of Fig. 2. The section between two adjacent valleys is seen as one heart beat. The reason why HR can be obtained from the difference result is related to heart's working mode. In a heartbeat cycle, the duration of systole is much less than diastole. Heart beat causes periodic change of the volume of vessel and then causes periodic change of the feature values we compute. As a result, the absolute value of difference during systole is more than diastole.

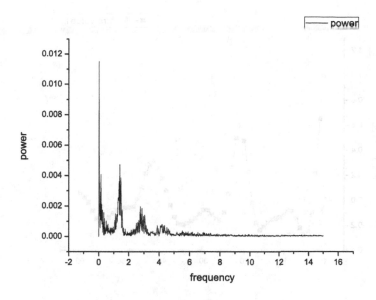

Fig. 4. The FFT result of data in Fig. 2

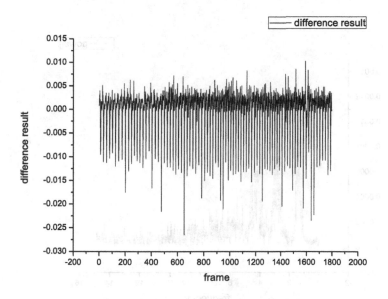

Fig. 5. The FD result of data in Fig. 2

AC can also be used to process the difference result and get the duration of one heartbeat cycle. The processed result of Fig. 5 is showed in Fig. 6. The HR obtained from Fig. 6 agrees with the result from Fig. 3. Fig. 7 shows the FFT result of data in Fig. 5. And when frequency is 1.406Hz in the range [0.4,2.0], the power is maximal.

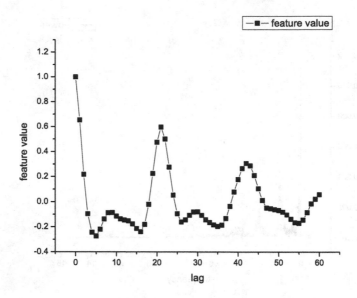

Fig. 6. The FDAC result of data in Fig. 2. (The AC result of data in Fig. 5.)

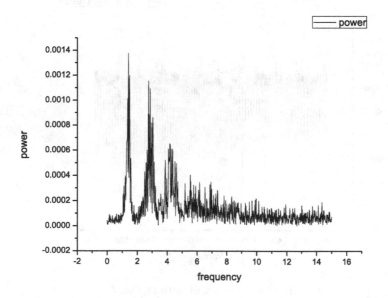

Fig. 7. The FD and FFT result of data in Fig. 2. (The FFT result of data in Fig. 5.)

3 Results and Discussion

There were 3 subjects and 6 tests for each one. The time of test was random in a certain day and in a well-lit environment. Manual peak detection was used on the time series, and the result was sufficiently seen as the real HR. In order to get spectral distribution of heartbeat cycle, the sequence which come from the time series subtract the mean value was processed by FFT. The difference result was processed by FFT as well. AC and FDAC were used to get the duration of heartbeat cycle.

Table 1. The calculated HR and corresponding relative errors

subject	Real HR	HR via FFT	Relative error (FFT)	HR via FD and FFT	Relative error (FD and FFT)	HR via AC	Relative error (AC)	HR via FDAC	Relative error (FDAC)
1	75	76	1.33%	76	1.33%	75	0.00%	75	0.00%
1	84	84	0.00%	84	0.00%	86	2.38%	86	2.38%
1	91	91	0.00%	91	0.00%	90	1.10%	90	1.10%
1	89	89	0.00%	89	0.00%	90	1.12%	90	1.12%
1	94	91	3.19%	91	3.19%	95	1.06%	95	1.06%
1	86	85	1.16%	85	1.16%	86	0.00%	86	0.00%
2	74	74	0.00%	74	0.00%	75	1.35%	75	1.35%
2	72	74	2.78%	74	2.78%	72	0.00%	72	0.00%
2	79	81	2.53%	81	2.53%	86	8.86%	78	1.27%
2	70	70	0.00%	70	0.00%	69	1.43%	69	1.43%
2	62	61	1.61%	61	1.61%	62	0.00%	62	0.00%
2	73	76	4.11%	76	4.11%	75	2.74%	75	2.74%
3	66	66	0.00%	66	0.00%	67	1.52%	67	1.52%
3	63	61	3.17%	62	1.59%	62	1.59%	60	4.76%
3	66	65	1.52%	65	1.52%	72	9.09%	66	0.00%
3	69	61	11.59%	61	11.59%	67	2.90%	64	7.25%
3	75	80	6.67%	80	6.67%	–	–	78	4.00%
3	79	76	3.80%	76	3.80%	78	1.27%	78	1.27%

Table 2. The percentage of correct estimations of actual HR

FFT	FD and FFT	AC	FDAC
88.89%	88.89%	83.33%	94.44%

Table 1, in which the corresponding relative errors were calculated, shows the final result. If the relative error was clear and less than 5%, and then the corresponding test was qualified. For each method, the number of qualified tests divided by the number of total tests was considered as the accuracy of the measurement. Table 2 shows the percentage of correct estimations of actual HR. Table 1 and 2 shows the high accuracy of the methods we utilized. However, there were some unsatisfactory results. For example, the spectral analysis results of the 4th test of subject 3 had large relative error. In the 5th test of subject 3, the result from AC has no clear result, owing to we were not be able to find a explicit peak in the corresponding curve. Table 2 shows that the FDAC method obtained the best result among other three methods for measuring HR (94.44%).

In general, results of spectral analysis, AC and FDAC were satisfactory. Most of the results are accurate enough that verified the practicability of our proposed methods.

For a time series, which have n elements, the time complexity of FD is $O(n)$. If lag is k, the time complexity of AC is $O(n)$. We set the value of k ranges from 0 to h, the overall time complexity of FDAC is

$$O((h+2)*n) \tag{5}$$

In our test, no matter how the size of time series changes the value of h is invariable. Therefore, the method takes $O(n)$ time as compared to $O(n \log n)$ for FFT. Nonetheless, these measurement are sensitive about stability and regularity of the raw time series. The subject should stay in a good environment and keep still as far as possible.

Because of the advantages of FD and AC , it can be applied to measure RR, HR from ECG and other vital signs that can be described as periodic time series. Many studies have found that there is a strong correlation between pulse wave velocity (PWV) and BP. For example, Steptoe A et al. have studied the correlation between PWV and mean arterial pressure (MAP) and proved that PWV can be an index of BP change [9]. The study about using FD and AC to analyse this correlation has been put into our plan.

4   Conclusion

In this paper, we proposed a new approach for HR detection. This approach relies on FD and AC. Although it requires some level of body surface contact, it does not cause any physical discomfort. The study result shows that the approach has low time complexity, low cost and better accuracy. It contributes to the fields of non-invasive health state detection.

Acknowledgments. This work is supported by Cuiying Grant of China Telecom, Gansu Branch(grant no. lzudxcy-2013-3), Science and Technology Planning Project of Chengguan District, Lanzhou grant no. 2013-3-1) and Scientific Research Foundation for the Returned Overseas Chinese Scholars, State Education Ministry (grant no. 44th).

References

1. Fitbit Inc., http://www.fitbit.com
2. Moves, http://www.moves-app.com
3. Instant Heart Rate, http://www.azumio.com/apps/heart-rate/
4. AliveCor Heart Monitor, http://www.alivecor.com/home
5. Chekmenev, S.Y., Rara, H., Farag, A.A.: Non-contact, wavelet-based measurement of vital signs using thermal imaging. In: The First International Conference on Graphics, Vision, and Image Processing (GVIP), Cairo, Egypt (2005)
6. Pursche, T., Krajewski, J., Moeller, R.: Video-based heart rate measurement from human faces. In: 2012 IEEE International Conference on Consumer Electronics (ICCE). IEEE (2012)
7. Poh, M.-Z., McDuff, D.J., Picard, R.W.: Advancements in noncontact, multiparameter physiological measurements using a webcam. IEEE Transactions on Biomedical Engineering 58(1), 7–11 (2011)
8. Box, G.E.P., Jenkins, G.M., Reinsel, G.C.: Time series analysis: forecasting and control. John Wiley & Sons (2013)
9. Steptoe, A., Smulyan, H., Gribbin, B.: Pulse wave velocity and blood pressure change: calibration and applications. Psychophysiology 13(5), 488–493 (1976)

Visual Analysis for Type 2 Diabetes Mellitus – Based on Electronic Medical Records

Xi Meng[1] and Ji-Jiang Yang[2]

[1] Department of Public Security Intelligence Science,
People' Public Security University of China, Beijing 100038, China
ximeng24@aliyun.com
[2] RIIT, Tsinghua University, Beijing 100084, China
TNList, Tsinghua University, Beijing 100084, China
yangjijiang@tsinghua.edu.cn

Abstract. A multidimensional-scaling approach is proposed to analyze the main symptoms of T2DM. Based on 200 Type 2 diabetes patients' electronic medical records, the terms which were used to described symptoms in the records and their co-occurring query terms were analyzed. A distanced-based similarity measure was used to calculate the proximity of terms to one and another based on their co-occurrences in the 200 medical records. After the calculation of the distance between each two keywords, a visual clustering of groups of terms was conducted. Each terms distribution within each visual configuration showed the most common symptoms of Type 2 diabetes such as Foam in Urine, Intermittent Dizziness, Hyperlipemia, Feeble, Diuresis etc; however it also showed some hidden relations behind our cognition.

Keywords: T2DM, visualization, visual analysis, co-word, MDS.

1   Introduction

Diabetes mellitus is a group of metabolic disease characterized by hyperglycemia resulting from defects in insulin secretion, insulin action, or both [1]. The patients' various organs are often dysfunction under Diabetes mellitus. One category of DM is Type 2 diabetes mellitus (T2DM), which is much more prevalent and common. It is hard to detect T2DM in people's daily life because its clinical symptoms are not very salient. Therefore, research and development of T2DM has received growing attention in the medical field. Studies have shown that Type 2 diabetes has recently emerged as a major global health problem. Over the past three decades, the number of people with diabetes mellitus has more than doubled globally, making it one of the most important public health challenges to all nations [2]. T2DM are increasingly observed among children, adolescents and younger adults. The symptoms of T2DM are embedded in a very complex group of genetic and epigenetic systems. The Diabetes Prevention Program Research Group reported how a lifestyle-intervention program or the administration of metformin would prevent or delay the development of diabetes. They conclude that the lifestyle intervention was more effective than metformin [3]. Frank B. Hu researched the T2DM in Asian countries. He claimed that

X. Zheng et al. (Eds.): ICSH 2014, LNCS 8549, pp. 160–170, 2014.
© Springer International Publishing Switzerland 2014

abdominal, central obesity is creating the widespread "metabolically obese" phenotype. Poor nutrition in utero and in early life plus over-nutrition in later life also contributes to the current diabetes epidemic in Asian populations [4].Although many factors including family genetic disease, smoking history and other causes contribute to the etiology of T2DM, there is no research to verify the noteworthy clinical symptoms which are involved in T2DM.

In this study, the relationships among various kinds of T2DM symptoms are analyzed. Multi-dimensional scaling analysis (MDS) method is employed to project high dimensional data into low dimensional space to better visualize the relationship among those symptoms. The performance of the proposed method is evaluated by two indicators of SPSS and the results suggest that the proposed method can display the relationships of T2DM symptoms and reveal some subtle connections between them.

2   Related Research

The main symptoms of T2DM can be explored in many ways: using surveys and interviews with clinical professionals, or by filtering information from popular medical websites, etc. Among them, electronic medical records analysis, a patient-centered approach, plays a very important role in understanding patient's description of experienced symptoms. Medical record is a legal document provides a chronicle of a patient's medical history and care [5]. Medical record, sometime also refers to health record or medical chart, is used interchangeably to describe the systematic documentation of a single patient's medical history and care across time within one particular health care provider's jurisdiction [6]. Medical record contains variety of types of "notes" entered over time by health care professionals, recording observations and administration of drugs and therapies, orders for the administration of drugs and therapies, test results, x-rays, reports, etc. One of the key constituent parts of medical records is the patient's symptoms description.

Many researches are using medical records as data sources [7-9]. In order to gain some understanding of wellbeing in patients following open heart surgery, researchers tried to explore health-care professionals' medical records by a content analysis [10]. In another research, researchers considered that documentation of expressions of decreased wellbeing perceived by HCPs in their communication with patients is an important piece of the puzzle, as it forms a basis both for decisions and for understanding the patient's overall health situation [11].The medical records system employed at the hospital was usually based on medical terms in order to make it easy to read and find information. The terms used in medical records are medical vocabulary and terminology, and can represent the salient attributions of the disease. Medical records analysis, which refers to the study of patients 'symptoms, has attracted the attention of researchers for many years. Medical records analysis can reveal first-hand and real-world patients' information. It enables researchers to better understand patients 'detailed symptoms and reflect the complexity of undergoing symptoms.

Using visualization method to reveal the hidden relationships among patients' data from the medical records is not a new endeavor. Along with the development of the related researches in the field, visualization method has become a complex systematical project that covers various kinds of data processing methods. In this study, the co-word analysis with MDS and clustering techniques is selected as the data processing tool to analyze the main causes of T2DM. Co-word analysis method was first proposed in the 1970's. It has been widely applied in many research fields. Co-word analysis is used to determine the clustering of closely related entries. It is a powerful method in discovering relationships among research objects and revealing hidden connections that may be not obvious [12]. The hypothesis of co-word analysis are: (1) Two entries appear in the same document also illustrates the correlations of these two themes [13]; (2) The co-occurrence, which aims to obtain hierarchical clustering based on similarity measure [14], is consistent with the common research subjects, objectives, and interests.. Although co-word analysis on subjects' medical records is challenging, it is meaningful and reliable.

Multidimensional Scaling (MDS) is one of the most popular techniques that conducts relatedness measurements. It has been widely used in data visualization in many research fields. MDS refers to a broad class of exploratory data tools that display the structure of high dimensional distance-like data as a geometrical picture. It maps the N objects data into a p-dimensional vector space. The mapping is chosen such that inter-vector distances approximate the given pairwise dissimilarities among the N objects. Compared with other visualization methods, MDS has its own advantages. The data used in MDS analysis is relatively free of any distributional assumptions; it can handle various types of data including ordinal, interval, and ratio-level data [15].Researchers proposed to visualize how close or similar the new patient is to others in the database by a modified multidimensional scaling technique that focuses on the correct positioning of the new patient in the visualization [16].

As the healthcare industry is now facing the challenge from the "big data" analysis, clustering techniques shows its unique advantage in medical records research field, where the traditional methods may fail to manage such large scale and complex data samples. By examining the clustering of patient records for chronic diseases, researchers are able to facilitate a better construction of care plan for the patient [17]. Mining medical record has a very close relationship with medical records clustering. The clinical data from medical record was considered to have a great research potential [18].Generally speaking, information visualization methods can be used for object/Subject clustering analysis. The visual presentation can clearly illustrate object relationship in a two or three-dimensional space. It helps people to observe multiple perspectives of relationships among objects in a vivid way. It demonstrates not only connections among the observed objects but also contexts where the objects are located and how they are connected.

In the research field of T2DM, there are few researches that focused on exploring the relationship between each of the symptoms and exploring if there is any hidden factor that causes the T2DM. As our lifestyle becomes more and more diversified, it is likely that people suffer from T2DM abruptly. Research on revealing the relationship of T2DM symptoms not only provides references or young and new clinical doctors when making decisions, but also helps patients learn more information of this aspect.

The goals of this study are:

- What are the main symptoms related to T2DM, especially hidden ones?
- What are the relationships between the symptoms?
- Better understand how usually patients descript their T2DM symptoms; therefore verify whether there is a general knowledge gap exist in public.

- Help young and new doctors to understand some easily ignored T2DM causes and provide them some references.
- Offer useful information for T2DM researchers. The findings may expand their research thinking and horizon.
- This study uses a visualization method to reveal the symptoms of T2DM.The primary aim of this study is to dig the hidden symptoms of T2DM, illustrate the relationships and shed light on the understanding of T2DM.

3   Research Method Description

3.1   Data Source

200 medical records from patients who had T2DM over a 1-year period dated from 2012-2013 had been collected for the experiment. Based on the confidentiality of medical records, all patients' names were dismissed in this research. Each of these patients had been diagnosed several times and the medical record was assigned a unique diagnosed code.

3.2   Term Extraction

Terms are extracted from the main body of medical records. These terms that related to symptoms or histories were revealed and identified in visual term analysis. Then all the extracted terms formed a term master file. All terms are filtered and synonyms, plurals and abbreviations of raw terms are normalized. Specifically, in the extraction process, the terms extracted from the records will be kept only if it does not match the stop word list. The stop word includes, but not limited to the most common, grammatical, and related words, such as "a", "the", "and", etc. In this manuscript, the stop word refers to subject stop word. Different from that of common stop words, the subject stop word are those key word frequently used in a Subject specific domain. In other words, in this specific domain, almost every document are related to these key word, thus they cannot be used as an index entry. For instance, in a medical record, "medical" can't be included in the subject terms since the term doesn't have its specific reference.

Therefore, all the terms became the standard entry terms. The term cleansing process enhanced the quality of analyzed unit and made sure the terms related to the same concept excluded. Next, the frequency of each term was tallied. In order to achieve a plausible clustering analysis result, a frequency cut-off point was set to eliminate the term which were less related. Low-frequency terms which make no sense were also cut off. The reason to process terms under this procedure is that the lower the term frequency, the less relevant the term is to the T2DM, and vice versa.

3.3   Term-Term Proximity Matrix

The term master file can be converted to a term-document matrix as shown in equation (1). Each row of Matrix_1 represents the subject terms filtered from T2DM medical records while each column represents the corresponding medical record documents.

$$\text{Matrix\_1} = \begin{bmatrix} d_{11} & d_{12} & \cdots & d_{1m} \\ d_{21} & d_{22} & \cdots & d_{2m} \\ \vdots & \vdots & \ddots & \vdots \\ d_{n1} & d_{n2} & \cdots & d_{nm} \end{bmatrix}, \tag{1}$$

In Equation (1), n is the number of the subject terms which are filtered from medical records, m is the number of the T2DM medical records (in this research, m=200), d_{nm} represents the frequency of term n in medical record document m. The first matrix is an $n \times m$ matrix.

Each term- document matrix was needed to be converted to a new term-term matrix. The distance between each term was calculated based on a similarity measure. To conduct the visualization of subject terms, the proximity of each two terms was calculated and a similarity measure was selected to measure similarity between each two terms in the Equation (1). There are many similarity measures available to proceed the matrix, such as the Consine measure, Jacard measure and the Distance-based measure. Each similarity measure has its own advantages and disadvantages and this varies with the selected data sets [19]. It is worth noting that the selection of different measure similarities didn't change the constitutive relations of each two terms. In this research, a pilot study was conducted to select the similarity measure and the distance-based measure was selected to normalize the matrix. The distance-based similarity measure is defined as follows:

$$S(t_i, t_j) = \frac{1}{c^{\delta(t_i, t_j)}} \tag{2}$$

Where $c = 1.4$ in this study. t_i and t_j are two terms. And δ is a variable which is the distance of each two terms.

$$\delta = \left[(t_{1i} - t_{1j})^2 + (t_{2i} - t_{2j})^2 + \cdots + (t_{mi} - t_{mj})^2 \right]^{1/2}, \\ m = 1, 2, \ldots 200. \tag{3}$$

In Equation (2), $S(t_i, t_j)$ is the proximity of term i and j. t_{mi} and t_{mj} are the cells of the matrix defined in Equation (1). What we can observe from Equation (3) is that δ decreases with the two key words co-occurrence number increases. This suggests that these two key words have a high similarity. In MDS spectrum, this appears as these two key words have a small Euclidean distance.

The generated term-term matrix(Equation (4), which provides the proximity between each two terms, is defined as follow. The proximity between two terms is the result of dimension reduction of the highly dimensional space term-term relationship defined by Equation(1),(2)and (3).

$$\text{Matrix\_2} = \begin{bmatrix} d_{11} & d_{12} & \cdots & d_{1m} \\ d_{21} & d_{22} & \cdots & d_{2m} \\ \vdots & \vdots & \ddots & \vdots \\ d_{m1} & d_{m2} & \cdots & d_{mm} \end{bmatrix}, \tag{4}$$

Notice that the similarity between one term and itself is always equal to 1, then:

$$b_{kk} = 1, \quad 1 \le k \le m \tag{5}$$

Other cells' definitions are shown in Equation (6).

$$b_{ij} = S(t_i, t_j), \quad i \ne j, \quad 1 \le i, j \le m \tag{6}$$

Since the proximity between term A and term B is equal to the proximity between term B and term A, the matrix is an $m \times m$ symmetric matrix, therefore, $b_{ij} = b_{ji}$ always holds.

3.4   MDS Analysis

Multidimensional scaling (MDS) refers to a set of methods that discovering "hidden" structures in multidimensional data. Based on a proximity matrix derived from variables measured on objects as input entity, these distances are mapped on a lower dimensional (typically two or three dimensional) spatial representation [20]. MDS was chosen for this study because it is reliable and robust enough to process different types of data input. It provides visual clustering analysis for small- to medium-sized data sets and this characteristic fits well the nature of T2DM medical records used in this study. There are two indicators in MDS analysis to show the quality of results: the stress value, and the squared correlation index (RSQ). Analysis result with a stress value less than 0.10 and RSQ value more than 0.90 is usually considered reliable and plausible. A low stress value and/or high RSQ value represents low dimensionality of a data set and close associations among projected objects.

4   Research and Discussion

4.1   Term Frequency Analysis

There were totally 200 medical records of T2DM, so term extraction was applied to the 200 medical records. This extraction generated 2010 terms, which averaged about 10 terms per medical record. Then these 2010 terms were merged by regularizing into a list of 31 terms. For example, the term "marasmus" and "Weight loss" were merged into "weight loss". In like manner, "Polyphagia" and "easy to hungry". If patients' mother or father or cousin suffered DM, investigators used "family DM" to describe it. Besides that, Investigators deleted some extracted terms since frequency of these terms were low which illustrated that they were relevant less of main causes. These deleted terms included pyelonephritis, appendectomy, bitter taste .This merged list of 31 terms, known as the term master file, results of the MDS analysis showed that there were 31 related terms that extracted from 200 T2DM medical records.

The frequencies of the 31 terms which were filtered from medical records were ranked in descending order and kept in the master file（table1）. Based on the 31 terms, a 31*31 term-term occurrence matrix was produced.

Then, the matrix was put into SPSS to conduct clustering analysis which enable people to observe the inner relationships between each term and have a deep understanding of which symptoms are the crucial to T2DM.

Table 1. Term frequency

Terms	Frequency	Terms	Frequency
Weight loss	59	Chronic cholecystitis	44
Inappetency	57	Coolness Of Extremities	39
Hyperlipidemia	57	Foam Urine	39
Polydipsia	57	High Blood Pressure	39
Family diabetes	55	Blurring Of Vision	36
Urorrhagia	55	Fatty Liver	33
Intermittent Dizziness	54	Cerebral Embolism	33
Feeble	53	Coronary Heart	33
Smoking	52	Drink	25
Limbs tingling	51	Palpitate	25
Lower extremity weakness	45	Fractura	23
Dry mouth	45	Osteoarthritis	23
Cereral insufficiency	44	Frequent Urination at Night	22
Parents of hypertension	44	Osteoporosis	22
Reflux Esophagitis	44	Hyperhidrosis	22
Polyphagia	44		

4.2   Subject Term Clustering

Figure 1 shows MDS analysis of the 31 terms and table 2 shows the terms that every cluster included. In order to display the inner structure of the causes, every cluster showed in figure1 was coded from C1 to C9.Since it is mentioned that Stress value

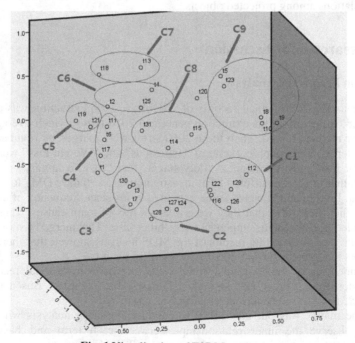

Fig. 1. Visualization of T2DM symptoms

and RSQ are two indicators that guarantee the reliability and validity of the analysis result, researchers need to inspect the two indicators in this study. The Stress value is 0.02863 and RSQ is 0.99790. It is in the range of acceptable.

It can be observed from Cluster1 that it mainly described the most notable symptoms of T2DM. Form in urine is one of the clinical symptoms of DM, but it can't diagnose DM only from this symptom. There are other typical symptoms. A lot of people with diabetes often suffer hyperlipemia as well and clinical consider it as the secondary disease in diabetes. Besides that, DM is often associated with intermittent dizziness, feeble and diuresis.

Cluster2 reveals that increased thirst (polydipsia) and hunger (polyphagia) usually accompany T2DM patients. They are the two of three main signs of diabetes. Besides that, t24 (Parents-Of-Hypertension) also appears in Cluster2. Diabetes is a kind of hereditary disease. People who have relatives with diabetes have much higher incidence to suffer diabetes.

Table 2. Nine clusters of T2DM symptoms

Clusters	Terms
C1	t12: Foam in Urine)
	t16: Intermittent Dizziness
	t22: Hyperlipemia
	t26: Feeble
	t29: Diuresis
C2	t27: Polydipsia
	t28: Polyphagia
	t24: Parents-Of-Hypertension
C3	t3: Frequent Urination at Night
	t7: Weight Loss
	t30: Hidrosis
C4	t1: Fatty Liver
	t11: Inappetency
	t6: Smoke
	t17: Family Diabetes
C5	t19: Osteoporosis
	t21: Osteoarthrosis
C6	t2: Drink
	t4: Palpitate
	t25: Reflux Esophagitis
C7	t13: Cerebral Embolism
	t18: Coronary Heart Disease
C8	t14: Cerebral insufficiency
	t15: Dry Mouth
	t31: Chronic Cholecystitis
C9	t5: Lower Extremity Weakness
	t8: Limbs Tingling
	t9: Coolness of Extremities
	t10: Blurring of Vision
	t23: High Blood Pressure

Cluster3 demonstrates that in the process of the development of diabetes, abnormal sweating is an important body signal of the complications of diabetes. Excessive sweating is accompanied by weight loss and sometimes results in excessive urge to urinate at night which is called "Hidrosis".

The theme of Cluster4 focuses on the association between fatty liver and diabetes. Patients with diabetes have a high prevalence of liver disease and patients with liver disease have a high prevalence of diabetes [21]. One of The common symptoms of fatty livers is inappetence. Another independent risk factor for diabetes is smoking which is harmful to both diabetes and fatty liver.

The theme of Cluster5 can be characterized into the joint disorders in terms of the complications of diabetes. Joint disorders tend to get mentioned less than the likes of retinopathy and kidney disease but some of the conditions can be serious [22]. The symptoms that Cluster 5 included develop subtle and can be hard to notice until "fragility fracture" happens.

Cluster 6 is mainly about Diabetic autonomic neuropathy and a series of reactions that the disease caused. Diabetic autonomic neuropathy is a common complication of diabetes mellitus and affects every segment of the gastrointestinal tract [23]. Especially, reflux esophagitis problems are more common and severe in T2DM patients. Reflux esophagitis can cause Palpitate. In Treato.com, there are 0.53% of the posts (40 posts) that mention Esophagitis also mention Palpitations [24]. Even though the percentage is quite low, it strongly demonstrates a series of symptoms which are caused by T2DM. In addition to Palpitation, T2DM patients with drink history are usually associated with these symptoms.

Cluster7 refers to the theme of cardiovascular and cerebral vascular diseases. Researchers even regarded T2DM as a "coronary heart disease equivalent" [25]. Cluster8 underlines that T2DM gives rise to cerebral insufficiency and accompanies symptoms of dry mouth. According to the statistical data of a personalized health information website "eHealthMe", due to 4th April 2014, ,397 people who have type 2 diabetes mellitus are studied. Among them, 46 (0.06%) have Chronic Cholecystitis. They amount to 0.06% of all the 77,088 people who have Chronic Cholecystitis on eHealthMe [26].

Long-term complications of diabetes include retinopathy with potential loss of vision; peripheral neuropathy with risk of foot ulcers, amputation, and Charcot joints [27]. The theme of C9 is relevant to the neuropathy which makes nerve degeneration. Patients experience hands and feet numbness, insensitive, foot deformation that make the foot easy to be damaged.

5   Conclusion

T2DM is associated with long-term damage and dysfunction of eyes, livers, nerves, heart and blood vessels. The clinical symptoms of T2DM show its diversity and uncertainty. Common symptoms of marked T2DM include polyuria, polydipsia, polyphagia and weight loss. Through visualization analysis of electronic medical records from clinical, some long-term complications of T2DM take the form of clustering including neuropathy with risk of joint disorders, autonomic neuropathy causing gastrointestinal, cardiovascular symptoms and other organs dysfunction. Some internal relations between symptoms are shown in the visual display. It helps us to observe some subtle connections between T2DM and symptoms. For instance, a weak connection between reflux esophagitis and T2DM is displayed. Even it was limited by the scale of data, researchers succeeded in visualizing the hidden causes and their relationships through MDS. This study identified and analyzed what the main symptoms are related to T2DM, especially hidden ones and the relationships between them.

The information visualization method like MDS is a powerful technique to mine the internal relationship which is hidden in the medical records. The visualization space provides the possibility of observing the research objects in 3D space. Using MDS method to analyze electronic medical records is a meaningful way to help better understand how usually patients descript their T2DM symptoms; verify whether there is a general knowledge gap exists in public; instruct young and new doctors to understand some easily ignored T2DM causes and provide them some references.

Future research will aim to expand the data scale and add new analysis topic to diabetes domain, hoping to provide more valuable analysis result.

References

1. American Diabetes Association. Diagnosis and classification of diabetes mellitus. J. Diabetes Care, 31(suppl. 1), 55–60 (2008)
2. Chen, L., Magliano, D.J., Zimmet, P.Z.: The worldwide epidemiology of type 2 diabetes mellitus present and future perspectives. J. Nature Reviews Endocrinology 8(4), 228–236 (2012)
3. Diabetes Prevention Program Research Group. Reduction in the incidence of type 2 diabetes with lifestyle intervention or metformin. N. Engl. J. Med. 346(6), 393–403 (February 7, 2002)
4. Hu, F.B.: Globalization of Diabetes: The role of diet, lifestyle, and genes. Diabetes Care 34(6), 1249–1257 (2011)
5. http://www.purdue.edu/push/appointments/recordreleasing. shtml (April 5, 2014)
6. Wikipedia, http://en.wikipedia.org/wiki/Medical_record#cite_note-1 (April 5, 2014)
7. Wang, S.J., Middleton, B., Prosser, L.A., et al.: A cost-benefit analysis of electronic medical records in primary care. J. The American Journal of Medicine 114(5), 397–403 (2003)
8. Wei, W.Q., Tao, C., Jiang, G., et al.: A high throughput semantic concept frequency based approach for patient identification: a case study using type 2 diabetes mellitus clinical notes. In: AMIA Annual Symposium Proceedings, pp. 857–861. American Medical Informatics Association (2012)
9. Cascade, E., Marr, P., Winslow, M., et al.: Conducting research on the Internet: medical record data integration with patient-reported outcomes. Journal of Medical Internet Research 14(5) (2012)
10. Karlsson, A.K., Lidell, E., Johansson, M.: Health-care professionals' documentation of wellbeing in patients following open heart surgery: a content analysis of medical records. J. Journal of Nursing Management 21(1), 112–120 (2013)
11. Adamsen, L., Tewes, M.: Discrepancy between patients' perspectives, staff's documentation and reflections on basic nursing care. J. Scandinavian Journal of Caring Sciences 14(2), 120–129 (2000)

12. Callon, M.: Pinpointing industrial invention: An exploration of quantitative methods for the analysis of patents. In: Callon, M., Law, J., Rip, A. (eds.) Mapping the Dynamics of Science and Technology: Sociology of Science in the Real World, pp. 163–188. Macmillan Press, London (1986)

13. Cambrosio, A., Limoges, C., Courtial, J.P., Laville, F.: Historical scientometrics? Mapping over 70 years of biological safety research with co-word analysis. J. Scientometrics 27, 119–143 (1993)

14. Braam, R.R., Moed, H.F., van Raan, A.F.J.: Mapping of science by combined co-citation and word analysis. II: Dynamical aspects. Journal of the American Society for Information Science 42, 252–266 (1991)

15. Zhang, J., Wolfram, D., Wang, P., et al.: Visualization of health-subject analysis based on query term co-occurrences. J. Journal of the American Society for Information Science and Technology 59(12), 1933–1947 (2008)

16. Klawonn, F., Lechner, W., Grigull, L.: Case-Centred multidimensional scaling for classification visualisation in medical diagnosis. In: Huang, G., Liu, X., He, J., Klawonn, F., Yao, G. (eds.) HIS 2013. LNCS, vol. 7798, pp. 137–148. Springer, Heidelberg (2013)

17. Saha, B., Pham, D.-S., Phung, D., Venkatesh, S.: Clustering patient medical records via sparse subspace Representation. In: Pei, J., Tseng, V.S., Cao, L., Motoda, H., Xu, G., et al. (eds.) PAKDD 2013, Part II. LNCS (LNAI), vol. 7819, pp. 123–134. Springer, Heidelberg (2013)

18. Jensen, P.B., Jensen, L.J., Brunak, S.: Mining electronic health records: towards better research applications and clinical care. J. Nature Reviews Genetics 13(6), 395–405 (2012)

19. Korfhage, R.R.: Information Storage and Retrieval. Wiley, New York (1997)

20. De Leeuw, J., Mair, P.: Multidimensional scaling using majorization: SMACOF in R.J. (2011)

21. Tolman, K.G., Fonseca, V., Dalpiaz, A., et al.: Spectrum of liver disease in type 2 diabetes and management of patients with diabetes and liver disease. J. Diabetes Care 30(3), 734–743 (2007)

22. http://www.diabetes.co.uk/diabetes-complications/diabetes-joint-pain-and-bones.html

23. Vinik, A.I., Maser, R.E., Mitchell, B.D., et al.: Diabetic autonomic neuropathy. J. Diabetes Care 26(5), 1553–1579 (2003)

24. http://treato.com/Esophagitis,Palpitations/?a=s

25. Juutilainen, A., Lehto, S., Rönnemaa, T., et al.: Type 2 Diabetes as a "Coronary Heart Disease Equivalent" An 18-year prospective population-based study in Finnish subjects. J. Diabetes Care 28(12), 2901–2907 (2005)

26. http://www.ehealthme.com/cs/type+2+diabetes+mellitus/cholecy stitis+chronic

27. American Diabetes Association. Diagnosis and classification of diabetes mellitus. J. Diabetes Care 31(suppl. 1), S55–S60 (2008)

A Preliminary Variable Selection Based Regression Analysis for Predicting Patient Satisfaction on Physician-Patient Cancer Prognosis Communication

Shuai Fang[1], Wenting Shi[1], Nan Kong[2], and Cleveland G. Shields[3]

[1] Department of Statistics, Purdue University, West Lafayette, IN, USA
{fang53,shi68}@purdue.edu
[2] Weldon School of Biomedical Engineering, Purdue University, West Lafayette, IN, USA
nkong@purdue.edu
[3] Department of Human Development and Family Studies, Purdue University,
West Lafayette, IN, USA
cgshields@purdue.edu

Abstract. We explore the use of variable selection methods to deal with high correlations among predicative variables (e.g., physician's voice tone and language certainty) for examining physician communication associated with prognosis discussion with cancer patients. Our main method is principal component analysis. The comparative results show its benefit in predicting patient satisfaction on the prognosis communication. This preliminary regression analysis is expected to offer insights into patient-centered communication strategy design, especially for cancer prognosis communication with end-stage patients.

Keywords: Patient centeredness, Variable selection, Principal component analysis, Patient Satisfaction, Cancer prognosis.

1 Introduction

Patient centeredness is identified as a core component of quality care [1]. It is defined as "health care that establishes a partnership among practitioners, patients, and their families (when appropriate) to ensure that decisions respect patients' wants, needs, and preferences and the patients have the education and support they need to make decisions and participate in their own care."[2]. Patient-centered care is supported by good physician-patient communication so that patients are treated as unique individuals rather than the illness is the strict focus [2,3,4,5]. The patient-centered approach in health care has been shown to help build a therapeutic alliance based on the patients' and the provider's perspectives and consequently improve patients' health and health care [3,4], [6,7,8] and reduce unnecessary medical spending [6], [9,10]. Unfortunately, many barriers exist to good communication. First and foremost, physicians often differ in communication proficiency, including varied listening skills and different views of symptoms and treatment effectiveness from their patients' [11]. Additional factors influencing patient centeredness and physician-patient communication

X. Zheng et al. (Eds.): ICSH 2014, LNCS 8549, pp. 171–180, 2014.
© Springer International Publishing Switzerland 2014

include: language barriers, racial and ethnic concordance between the patient and the physician, effects of disabilities on patients' health care experiences, as well as physicians' cultural competency.

Efforts to remove these possible impediments to patient centeredness are underway in the U.S. Department of Health and Human Services [12]. Meanwhile, in the academic field of health behavioral and communication, several human subject studies (e.g., [13]) have been conducted to examine physician-patient interactions and offer insights to guideline development for specific medical decision making processes. Much of the investigation was focused on designing measurement instruments of patient-centered communication and testing hypotheses on selected factors on the communication outcomes. While studies are available in the literature reporting descriptive statistics, correlation analyses, and multivariate regression analyses, none of the work, to our knowledge, has systematically applied regression and prediction techniques to a large set of attainable factors that could be potentially influencing to evaluate their impacts and interdependencies on the communication outcomes. In this paper, we report a preliminary study that applies variable section and develops regression models for patient satisfaction from the communication. In our work, we focused on examining physician communication associated with prognosis discussion with cancer patients. Our work is expected to help make better informed decisions on selecting physician's communication approach for engaging patients in cancer prognosis discussions. It will also offer insights into doing data-driven prospective research on shared medical decision making and investigating effective delivery of patient-centered care.

For our study, we acquired data from a pilot study, conducted by one of the authors, that examines the prognosis discussions during oncology visits. While guidelines exist for discussing prognosis with cancer patients [14,15], there is no firm evidence supporting any one approach [16]. It is well reported in the literature that both patient and physician factors affect prognosis discussion in medical encounters [17]. First, culture is likely to be a significant factor on prognosis communication. In general, cancer patients from western cultures tend to prefer acquiring knowledge on their diagnosis findings, prognosis, and probability of successfully treating their diseases [18,19]; but not all cultures endorse such a preference. As a result, physicians from non-western cultures may be more reluctant to disclose prognostic information than western physicians [20]. Furthermore, it is difficult in practice to determine whether a specific cancer patient really wants to know his or her prognosis. It is common for patients not to understand their prognosis, which may hinder them and their attending physicians in shared decision making. Other general findings in the literature only indicate that patients prefer a realistic and hopeful style when disclosing diagnosis and hope is conveyed partly by discussing all the treatment options [21].

Prognosis discussions are hampered by the different focuses of the patient and the physician. Patients tend to focus on the impact of cancer on their lives as well as their discomfort and pain, whereas physicians tend to focus on the illness, particularly on its progression and treatment. In the study from which we acquired the data, standard patients were employed for controlling patient characteristics and thus maintaining consistent delivery of messages on patients' desire about prognosis information. Based on a number of hypotheses from the previous studies, we selected three sets of physician controlled independent variables related to patient-centeredness. They were used to measure the carefulness of information gathering, voice tone used in the prognosis communication, and physician use of certainty language. We also included variables that quantify the prognosis discussion. The dependent variable is the average of standardized patient satisfaction measures, which serves as a proxy of the effectiveness in prognosis communication. More details on the predictive variables and outcome measure are given in Section 2.

The remainder of the paper is organized as follows. In Section 2, we describe our methods in both human subject study design and predictive model development. In Section 3, we report and discuss our comparative results. In Section 4, we conclude the paper by outlining the limitations of the work and future research directions.

2 Methods

2.1 Human Subject Study Design

Standard patients (SPs) were employed in a pilot human subject study (Shields et al. [13]) to realize more control for the variation in patient participation in the prognosis discussion. These SPs were actors trained to portray with high fidelity stage IV lung cancer patients who sought help for uncontrolled pain. They made unannounced visits to consenting physicians. This method has been extensively used in primary care research [22,23,24,25,26] but, to our knowledge, has not been used to examine oncology patient visits. We provide more details in the following.

Study Participants and Procedures. The pilot study recruited 46 physicians, 23 family physicians and 23 oncologists, through the Family Practice Research Network in a Midwestern state and through senior specialists at a regional medical center. The final sample consisted of 39 physicians, 20 family physicians and 19 oncologists, due to physician withdrawal and departure, as well as recording loss.

The relevant human subjects review boards approved the study. Three male SPs were trained to portray a patient with an advanced life-threatening illness with radiographic and laboratory evidence supporting the patient's complaint of severe pain. During each unannounced visit, each SP carried two concealed audio-recorders (one for backup). For the controlled physician-patient interaction during each visit, the SP was given a complete script that details the clinical and personal history responses to potential physician questions or actions. Weeks after the visit, the physician was asked whether suspected one of their patients to be an actor and asked to describe the patient.

The obtained audiotapes were reviewed by the study designer and the SPs were debriefed weekly to optimize their role fidelity. The role fidelity was assessed by rating each SP visit based on a coding checklist of twenty items, which encompassed the major dimensions of the role. Each dimension was assessed using a 1-5 Likert-type scale with 1 being *not portrayed at all* to 5 being *a very accurate portrayal of that part of the role*. With the assessment on each dimension, the overall percentage of adherence of SP to the role was assessed. A follow-up study in [27] also reported that the physicians suspected SPs in only 14% of the visits, a level found in similar studies (e.g., [28]).

Predictive Variables. Based on several hypotheses in the existing literature [13],[22],[27], we selected 13 predictive variables. The majority of them fall into four categories on eliciting/validating patient concerns, voice tone, physician use of certainty language, and assessment of prognosis communication. The first two categories are related to measuring patient-centered communication. Other variables include total interaction time, patient's word count, as well as physician's gender, age and occupation. Table 1 lists the descriptive statistics about these predictive variables. We explain them and their associated measurement instruments in the following.

Table 1. Predictive variables and descriptive statistics about them

Category	Variable Name	Characteristic	Oncologist			Family Physician		
			Mean	SD	Range	Mean	SD	Range
Eliciing/ Validating patient concerns	Elicit_val	Average score of 19 items of 1-5 scale	1.05	0.66	0.17– 2.33	1.42	0.65	0.42- 2.67
Voice tone	attentive	Average scores among four raters using 1-7 scale	3.92	0.90	2.5-5.5	3.75	0.88	1.75-5
	anxious		2.94	1.06	2-5	3	0.78	1-4
	hostile		2.22	0.88	1-5	2	0.77	1-4
Physician use of certainty in the lang.	P_WC	Integer word count	1394	984	410- 4249	1673	659	555- 2961
	youdying	Binary indict- or	0.61	0.50	{0,1}	0	0.44	{0,1}
Assessing prognosis communication	prog_sum	Aggregate score of items of 1-5 scale	11.72	7.30	0-27	7	6.18	0-23
	prog_freq	Integer	4.47	2.15	1-9	3	2.14	1-8
Miscellaneous	D_WC	Integer word count	1957	1150	486- 5290	1928	1213	728- 5394
	totaltime	Integer (in mins)	28.19	13.33	9.5-56	30	12.99	15-72.5
	Age	Integer	46.56	7.64	35-68	50	10.29	31-72
	Male	Binary indicator	0.72	0.46	{0,1}	1	0	{0,1}

Eliciting/Validating Patient Concerns. A list of 19 patient concerns was created and coded to measure the carefulness of the physician in gathering relevant information about the SP. These items implies whether physicians conducted preliminary information elicitation, further exploration, and validation to discussion topics such as mood/depression, family support, disease's impact on life, previous physicians, and scans done since diagnosis. Each item was quantified with a 1-5 scale and the average scores were reported. An item analysis was then conducted to eliminate several items. The final scale had a satisfactory level of coding reliability (i.e., Cronbach's alpha of

0.78 and the intraclass correlation coefficient was 0.88), indicating the coding differentiated cases, not coders. For more information on internal consistency, we refer to Cronbach [29].

Voice Tone. Three measures were used to characterize the physician's voice tone. They are anxious/attentive/hostile tones. A number of independent raters listened to the audio recordings and coded for the voice tone using a 1–7 scale in a manner similar to the Roter Interaction Analysis System (RIAS) [30]. For example, to measure attentiveness voice tone, each physician was rated on four separate items: warmth, concern, worry, and openness. The average was then taken. Again, the final scale had satisfactory internal consistency among the raters.

Physician Use of Certainty in the Language. Linguistic Inquiry and Word Count (LIWS), a text analysis program [31] was used to tally the amount and percentage of certainty words said by physicians in an encounter with SPs. LIWC uses words such as absolute, certain, clear, complete, confident, definite, and sure (see www.liwc.net for more information). Individuals who use more certainty-conveying words seek causal understandings [32], an important task for physician making diagnoses. However, because those who have a need for certainty tend to be less tolerant of ambiguity, they may curtail data gathering and engage in premature closure [33]. In addition, an indicator was recorded on whether the physician used phrases to strongly indicate the mortality possibility to SPs.

Assessing Prognosis Communication. Ten items were created to assess physicians' behaviors that communicate diagnostic information and treatment option (palliative care) that are likely to be offered to a stage IV lung cancer patient. The creation was based on the components of the SPIKES protocol for delivering bad news [14]. The coding for these items was similar to coding eliciting and validating in that they used the same physician response code. Nevertheless, they remain separate constructs because they coded very different communication behaviors. For each physician-patient interaction, once the ten items were quantified, we aggregated their values into a predictive variable that quantifies the depth with which prognosis was being discussed. Additionally, we recorded the number of times prognosis being discussed during each physician-patient interaction.

To summarize the above description, we have 1 predictive variable from the category of eliciting/validating patient concerns, 3 variables related to voice tone, 2 variables related to physician use of certainty in the language, and 2 variables related to assessing prognosis communication. In addition, we included 1 variable measuring the total physician-patient interaction time (in minutes), 1 variable measuring patient engagement by counting the words he/she spoke during the interaction, 3 variables indicating the

Table 2. Correlation table with selected variables

Variable	1	2	3	4	5
1 % of certainty words*	--				
2 eliciting/validating	.29	--			
3 anxious voice tone	.15	.39	--		
4 physician gender (F:0; M:1)	.01	.11	.13	--	
5 physician occupation (0: family physician; 1: oncologist)	.10	.10	.27	.10	--

*: instead of total account of the certainty words, we used percentage here

physician's age, gender (1 being *Male* and 0 being *Female*), and occupation (1 being *an oncologist* and 0 being *a family physician*). We conducted a preliminary correlational analysis. The results (see Table 2) indicated that most of the variables are significantly correlated. This motivates us to explore the use of variable selection techniques to systematically conduct regression analysis. As a preliminary study, we applied principal component analysis for variable feature and applied linear regression to the selected principal components. We also applied standard linear regression assisted by model selection for the comparison purpose.

Patient Satisfaction Outcome Measure. A post-visit questionnaire given to the SPs contained 5 sections. These sections measured (1) SP's perception on the physician's prognosis communication (HCCQ section with 5 questions); (2) SP's believe on how well the physician knows him/her (KNOW section with 4 questions); (3) how satisfied the SP is with the physician (sp_satisfied); (4) SP's trust on the physician (TRUST section with 7 questions); and (5) SP's overall trust on the physician (sp_overall_trust). All items in the HCCQ, KNOW, and TRUST sections were rated on a 1-5 scale and the sum scores were calculated. Variables sp_satisfied and sp_overall_trust were rated using a 1–6 scale with 1 being *completely satisfied couldn't be better* and 6 being *the complete opposite*, and a 0–10 scale with 0 being *not at all* and 10 being *completely trusting*, respectively. Table 3 lists all five variables from the five sections. Given the fact that these variables took different scales, we rescaled them to standard scores. We averaged the standard scores to get the final patient satisfaction outcome measure.

Table 3. Measures pertaining to patient satisfaction and descriptive statistics about them

Variable Name	Oncologist			Family Physician		
	Mean	SD	Range	Mean	SD	Range
hccq	10.78	3.21	6-18	10	3.73	6-17
know	9.83	2.81	5-16	10	3.13	5-16
sp_satisfied	2.61	1.14	1-5	3	1.20	1-5
trust	19.56	1.98	16-22	20	2.00	18-27
sp_overall_trust	7.44	1.38	5-9	6	2.02	3-10

2.2   Variable Selection and Regression Analysis

We applied regression analysis to develop predictive models and applied principal component analysis to alleviate the correlations among predictive variables. Principal component analysis (PCA) [34] is a valuable and commonly used multivariate technique for finding patterns and reducing correlations in data of high dimensions. PCA uses orthogonal transformation to convert a set of observations of possibly correlated variables into a set of values of linearly uncorrelated variables called *principal components*. The transform is defined in such a way that the first principal component has the largest possible variance, accounting for as much of the variability in the data as possible, and each succeeding component, in turn, has the largest variance possible under the constraint that it is orthogonal to (i.e., uncorrelated with) the preceding components. PCA is sensitive to the relative scaling of the original variables, so in our study we standardized all predictive variables. Once we selected the first few principal components, we identified their association with the predictive variables. Through some preliminary experiments, we concluded it would be reasonable to select 4 – 8 principal components. With such selection, about 70 – 90% of the variance in the data could be explained. Then we developed a regression model based on the selected principal components. In our actual implementation, we used the SAS FACTOR procedure with method = principal.

For comparison purpose, we applied generalized linear regression with all 13 predictive variables and performed model selection in the framework of general linear models. For model selection, we used the following criteria progressively: (1) higher adjusted R-square value; (2) smaller difference between Mallow's Cp statistic [35] and the number of model coefficients plus 1; (3) smaller Akaike information Criterion (AIC) measure [36]; and (4) Schwarz Bayesian information Criterion (SBC) measure [37]. We further conducted correlation tests to ensure no significant multicollinearity among the subset of variables selected. Lastly, we applied linear regression on the selected variables. To compare the developed models, we conducted leave-one-out cross validation that used 38 samples to build a regression model and tested it with the remaining sample. We calculated the sum of squares errors over all samples and compared the regression models with various error distribution assumptions. In our implementation, we used the SAS GLMSELECT procedure for the model selection and MATLAB for the leave-one-out cross-validation.

3   Results and Discussion

For the interest of space, we report the linear associations between the original predictive variables and the first 5 principal components selected (see Table 4). The table shows the correlation pattern among predictive variables as well as the association pattern between the predictive variables and the principal components. For example, variables *Elicit_val*, *attentive*, *P_WC*, *prog_sum*, *prog_freq*, *D_WC* should be grouped and they contribute significantly in explaining the variance in the data. The coefficients in the table also imply the linear functions that are used to convert the original predictive variables to the principal components. For example, for each physician, the converted value on PC1 = calculated as .635 × *Elcit_val* +.720 × *attentive* +...+ .018 × *Oncologist*. We then build a linear regression model of the standardized average satisfaction rating with the selected principal components being the predictive variables. Here we only assumed that the residuals are normally distributed.

Table 4. Principal component (PC) pattern table

Var.\PC	PC1	PC2	PC3	PC4	PC5
Elicit_val	**.635**	-.324	.272	.153	-.388
attentive	**.720**	-.152	-.089	-.373	.216
anxious	-.296	**.759**	.110	.019	-.115
hostile	-.568	**.587**	.247	.005	-.128
P_WC	**.641**	.059	.321	-.303	-.128
youdying	.267	**.800**	-.177	-.031	-.004
prog_sum	**.814**	.198	-.349	.198	-.200
prog_freq	**.762**	.146	-.436	.236	-.217
D_WC	**.583**	.294	.459	.077	.426
Totaltime	.478	.323	**.575**	.291	.283
Age	-.146	-.022	.216	**.748**	-.267
Male	-.058	.224	-.388	**.567**	.504
Oncologist	.018	.460	**-.654**	-.062	.092

For comparison, we performed model selection and selected 11 variables: *Elicit_val, attentive, anxious, hostile, prog_freq, prog_sum, Oncologist, Age, Totaltime, youdying, D_WC*. With correlation testing, we then found that *prog_freq* and *prog_sum* are highly correlated. We thus only included *prog_freq* in the variable set. In total, we had 10 variables. We then build a generalized regression model of the 10 variables with respect to the standardized patient satisfaction outcome and varied the assumption on the residual probability distribution.

Table 5 shows the comparison of the modeling methods based on the sum of square errors over all 39 samples. From the table, we observed that applying PCA in the framework of standard linear regression with normal distribution on the residual outperformed applying model selection in the framework of generalized linear regression. Note that we only reported the best SSE for the latter approach over various assumptions on the residual distribution. We also concluded that the relative superiority is insensitive to the number of principal components selected. With 5–7 principal components selected, the predictive modeling procedure empowered by PCA was quite robust. This further strengthened our belief that it is beneficial to carefully making variable selection among highly correlated predictive variables before applying regression analysis to predict cancer prognosis communication effectiveness outcomes.

Table 5. Predictive modeling procedure comparison

Predictive modeling method		SSE from cross-validation	Variance explained
PCA in standard linear regression	4 PCs selected	17.40	68.9%
	5 PCs selected	16.96	76.0%
	6 PCs selected	17.32	81.8%
	7 PCs selected	16.01	86.9%
	8 PCs selected	18.90	90.6%
GLM with model selection		26.88	n/a
GLM w/o model selection		35.51	n/a

4   Conclusions and Future Directions

Using a rigorous study design that controlled for patient-to-patient differences in prognosis communication, we examined physician behaviors associated with how satisfied the patient felt during the physician-patient interaction. Faced with the challenges that the collected data contain many highly correlated predictive variables but only of modest sample size, we explored the use of variable selection methods to empower the regression analysis and predictive model development. It is worth noting that this challenge is prevailing in health services research.

The small sample of physicians limits the extent to which our results can be generalized to other physicians. Although SPs have the advantage of controlling for variability in patient presentation, they also introduce the problem of first-visit bias [38]. Hence, future studies with larger samples are needed to replicate and confirm our findings. In addition, future studies are needed to identify potentially influencing features from the abundant communication sequence data with larger granularity, the majority of which is yet explored. Meanwhile, we will continue to explore the use of alternative variable and model selection procedures (e.g., correspondence analysis [39]) to further improve the predictive power. The ultimate goal is to assess whether changing physicians' mutable behaviors can lead to improved communication effectiveness in various shared medical decision making settings.

References

1. Institute of Medicine: Crossing the Quality Chasm: A New Health System for the 21st Century. National Academies Press, Washington DC (2001)
2. Institute of Medicine: Envisioning the National Health Care Quality Report. National Academies Press, Washington DC (2001)
3. Stewart, M., Brown, J.B., Donner, A., McWhinney, I.R., Oates, J., Weston, W.W., Jordan, J.: The Impact of Patient-Centered Care on Outcomes. J. Fam. Pract. 49(9), 796–804 (2000)
4. Anderson, E.B.: Patient-Centeredness: a New Approach. Nephrol. News Issues 16(12), 80–82 (2000)
5. Michie, S., Miles, J., Weinman, J.: Patient-Centeredness in Chronic Illness: What Is It and Does It Matter? Patient Educ. Couns. 51(3), 197–206 (2003)
6. Little, P., Everitt, H., Williamson, I., et al.: Observational Study of Effect of Patient Centeredness and Positive Approach on Outcomes of General Practice Consultations. BMJ 323(7318), 908–911 (2001)
7. DiMatteo, M.R.: The Role of the Physician in the Emerging Health Care Environment. West J. Med. 168(5), 328–333 (1998)
8. Beck, R.S., Daughtridge, R., Sloane, P.D.: Physician-Patient Communication in the Primary Care Office: A Systematic Review. J. Am. Board Fam. Pract. 15(1), 25–38 (2002)
9. Berry, L.L., Seiders, K., Wilder, S.S.: Innovations in Access to Care: A Patient-Centered Approach. Ann. Intern. Med. 139(7), 568–574 (2003)
10. Bechel, D.L., Myers, W.A., Smith, D.G.: Does Patient-Centered Care Pay Off? Jt. Comm. J. Qual. Improv. 26(7), 400–409 (2000)
11. Rhoades, D.R., McFarland, K.F., Finch, W.H., et al.: Speaking and Interruptions during Primary Care Office Visits. Fam. Med. 33(7), 528–532 (2001)
12. U.S. Department of Health and Human Services, Office of Minority Health: Think Cultural Health: Bridging the Health Care Gap through Cultural Competency Continuing Education Programs, http://www.thinkculturalhealth.hhs.gov
13. Shields, C.G., Coker, C.J., Poulsen, S.S., Doyle, J.M., Fiscella, K., Epstein, R.M., Griggs, J.J.: Patient-Centered Communication and Prognosis Discussion with Cancer Patients. Patient Educ. Couns. 77(3), 437–442 (2009)
14. Baile, W.R., Buckman, R., Lenzi, R., Glober, G., Beale, E.A., Kudelka, A.P.: SPIKES – a Six-Step Protocol for Delivering Bad News: Application to the Patients with Cancer. Oncologist 5(4), 302–311 (2000)
15. Clayton, J.M., Hancock, K.M., Butow, P.N., Tattersall, M.H.N., Currow, D.C.: Clinical Practice Guidelines for Communicating Prognosis and End-of-Life Issues with Adults in the Advanced Stages of a Life-Limiting Illness, and Their Caregivers. Med. J. Aust. 186(suppl. 12), S77–S108 (2007)
16. Hagerty, R.G., Butow, P.N., Ellis, P.M., Lobb, E.A., Pendlebury, S.C., Leighl, N., MacLeod, C., Tattersal, M.H.N.: Communicating with Realism and Hope: Incurable Cancer Patients' Views on the Disclosure of Prognosis. J. Clin. Oncol. 23(6), 1278–1288 (2005)
17. Steinmetz, D., Walsh, M., Gabel, L.L., Williams, P.T.: Family Physicians' Involvement with Dying Patients and Their Families. Attitudes, Difficulties, and Strategies. Arch. Fam. Med. 2(7), 753–760 (1993)
18. Cassileth, B.R., Zupkis, R.V., Sutton-Smith, K., March, V.: Information and Participation Preferences among Cancer Patients. Ann. Intern. Med. 92(6), 832–836 (1980)
19. Jenkins, V., Fallowfield, L., Saul, J.: Information Needs of Patients with Cancer: Results from a Large Study in UK Cancer Centers. Br. J. Cancer 84(1), 48–51 (2001)

20. Mitchell, J.L.: Cross-Cultural Issues in the Disclosure of Cancer. Cancer Pract. 6(3), 153–160 (1998)
21. Hagerty, R.G., Butow, P.N., Ellis, P.M., Dimitry, S., Tattersall, M.H.N.: Communicating Prognosis in Cancer Care: a Systematic Review of the Literature. Ann. Oncol. 16(7), 1005–1053 (2005)
22. Fiscella, K.M., Meldrum, S.M., Franks, P.M., Shields, C.G., Duberstein, P.P., McDaniel, S.H., Epstein, R.M.: Patient Trust: Is It Related to Patient-Centered Behavior of Primary Care Physicians? Med. Care 42(11), 1049–1055 (2004)
23. Epstein, R.M., Franks, P., Shields, C.G., Meldrum, S.C., Miller, K.N., Campbell, T.L., Fiscella, K.: Patient-Centered Communication and Diagnostic Testing. Ann. Fam. Med. 3(5), 415–421 (2005)
24. Tamblyn, R., Berkson, L., Dauphinee, W.D., Gayton, D., Grad, R., Huang, A., Isaac, L., McLeod, P., Snell, L.: Unnecessary Prescribing of NSAIDs and the Management of NSAID-Related Gastropathy in Medical Practice. Ann. Intern. Med. 127(6), 429–438 (1997)
25. Kravitz, R.L., Epstein, R.M., Feldman, M.D., Franz, C.E., Azari, R., Wilkes, M.S., Hinton, L., Franks, P.: Influence of Patients' Requests for Direct-to-consumer Advertised Antidepressants: a Randomized Controlled Trial. J. Am. Med. Assoc. 293(16), 1995–2002 (2005)
26. Peabody, J.W., Luck, J., Glassman, P., Dresselhaus, T.R., Lee, M.: Comparison of Vignettes, Standardized Patients, and Chart Abstraction a Prospective Validation Study of 3 Methods for Measuring Quality. J. Am. Med. Assoc. 283(13), 1715–1722 (2000)
27. Shields, C.G., Finley, M.A., Elias, C.M., Coker, C.J., Griggs, J.J., Fiscella, K., Epstein, R.M.: Pain Assessment: The Roles of Physician Certainty and Curiosity. Health Commun. 28(7), 740–746 (2013)
28. Franz, C.E., Epstein, R., Miller, K.N., Brown, A., Song, J., Feldman, M., Kelly-Reif, S., Kravitz, R.L.: Caught in the Act?: Prevalence, Predictors, and Consequences of Physician Detection of Unannounced Standardized Patients. Health Serv. Res. 41(6), 2290–2302 (2006)
29. Cronbach, L.J.: Coefficient Alpha and the Internal Structure of Tests. Psychometrika 16(3), 297–334 (1951)
30. Roter, D., Larson, S.: The Roter Interaction Analysis System (RIAS): Utility and Flexibility for Analysis of Medical Interactions. Patient Educ. and Couns. 46(4), 243–251 (2002)
31. Pennebaker, J.W., Chung, C.K., Ireland, M., Gonzales, A., Booth, R.J.: Operator's Manual: Linguistic Inquiry and Word Count. In: LIWC 2007 (2007), http://homepage.psy.utexas.edu/homepage/faculty/pennebaker/reprints/
32. Pennebaker, J.W., King, L.A.: Linguistic Styles: Language Use as an Individual Difference. J. Pers. Soc. Psychol. 77(6), 1296–1312 (2007)
33. Furnham, A., Ribchester, T.: Tolerance of Ambiguity: A Review of the Concept, Its Measurement and Applications. Current Psychology 14(3), 179–199 (1995)
34. Jolliffe, I.T.: Principal Component Analysis, 2nd edn. Springer Series in Statistics, vol. XXIX, p. 487. 28 illus. (2002); Bickel, P., Diggle, P., Fienberg, S.E., Gather, U., Olkin, I., Zeger, S. (series eds.)
35. Mallows, C.L.: Some Comments on Cp. Technometrics 15(4), 661–675 (1973)
36. Darlington, R.B.: Multiple Regression in Psychological Research and Practice. Psychological 69(3), 161–182 (1968)
37. Schwarz, G.: Estimating the Dimension of a Model. The Annals of Statistics 6(2), 461–464 (1978)
38. Beullens, J., Rethans, J.J., Goedhuys, J., Buntinx, F.: The Use of Standardized Patients in Research in General Practice. Family Practice 14, 58–62 (1997)
39. Le Roux, B., Rounet, H.: Geometric Data Analysis, From Correspondence Analysis to Structured Data Analysis. Kluwer, Dordrecht (2004)

Intelli-food: Cyberinfrastructure for Real-Time Outbreak Source Detection and Rapid Response

Matteo Convertino[1] and Craig Hedberg[2]

[1] Division of Environmental Health Sciences, & Health Informatics Program, Institute on the Environment, Institute for Engineering in Medicine, Food Safety Integrated Centers of Excellence, University of Minnesota Twin-Cities
[2] Division of Environmental Health Sciences, & Health Informatics Program, Food Safety Integrated Centers of Excellence, University of Minnesota Twin-Cities
http://www.tc.umn.edu/~matteoc/Welcome.html

Abstract. Foodborne diseases cause an estimated 48 million illnesses each year in the United States, including 9.4 million caused by known pathogens. Real time detection of cases and outbreak sources are important epidemic intelligence services that can decrease morbidity and mortality of foodborne illnesses, and allow optimal response to identify the causal pathways leading to contamination. For most outbreaks associated with fresh produce items, outbreak source detection typically occurs after the contaminated produce items have been consumed and are no longer in the marketplace. We developed a probabilistic model for real time outbreak source detection, prediction of outbreaks, and contamination-prone area mapping with the aim of developing a cyber-infrastructure to support this activity. The models inputs include environmental, trade and epidemiological dynamics. Because effective distance reliably predicts disease arrival times we estimate the distance of outbreak sources from spatio-temporal patterns of foodborne outbreaks. As a case study we consider the 2013 Cyclospora outbreaks in the USA that were related to contaminated fresh produce (cilantro and fresh salad mix) from Mexico. We are able to match case distributions related to both food commodities and determine their outbreak sources with an average accuracy of 0.93. Assuming a similar pattern of contamination for 2014, outbreak patterns can be similar or worse with an unchanged food trade that is likely. The study aims to provide a methodological framework to evaluate environmentally sensitive food contamination and assess interdependencies of socio-environmental factors causing contamination. We emphasize the linkage of patterns and processes, the positive role of uncertainty, and challenge the belief that information about the whole food supply chain is needed for traceback analysis to be useful for identifying likely sources. Our specific prediction strongly emphasizes the need for real-time surveillance to identify and respond to this pending outbreak.

Keywords: outbreak source, epidemic intelligence, outbreak patterns, effective distance, food trade.

X. Zheng et al. (Eds.): ICSH 2014, LNCS 8549, pp. 181–196, 2014.

1   Introduction

1.1   Foodborne Outbreaks and Limitations of Current Approaches to Foodborne Disease Surveillance

State, local and territorial public health departments have the primary responsibility for identifying and investigating foodborne disease outbreaks. Outbreak reports are compiled by the Center for Disease Control and Prevention (CDC) through a web-based program, the National Outbreak Reporting System (NORS). Despite efforts to improve coordination of surveillance on national and international levels through the use of laboratory-based systems such as PulseNet, differences in the efficiency of outbreak investigation and reporting by health agencies remain. Moreover, state and local health agencies frequently act independently of each other, creating difficulties in rapid detection and response to multi-state outbreaks. There is also lack of real-time computational tools for detecting outbreak sources [1–4]. Typically, health officials detect the outbreak source by combining epidemiologic and microbiologic data with food chain information obtained from food system stakeholders. This investigative approach is very time consuming and for most fresh produce-associated outbreaks, the precise detection of the source occurs after the implicated product has been exhausted from the marketplace [5]. This non-computationally based approach also has limited ability to predict potential future outbreaks, to provide information about the critical contamination-prone areas and in the surveillance system, and to deal with uncertainty in case, food trade, and microbiological data. An illustrative example of important limitations in the food surveillance system occurred in the summer of 2013 with a Cyclospora outbreak in USA [6].

1.2   Cyclospora Outbreaks and Case Study

Cyclospora infections cause watery, and sometimes explosive, diarrhea. The one-celled parasite can enter the body when people ingest contaminated food or water. Cyclospora has caused several multi-state outbreaks in the United States in the past decade, most of which have been traced back to fresh imported produce [6, 7]. In the USA, Cyclospora outbreaks have a typical summer peak that occurs following the distribution of contaminated fresh produce. Because the clinical illness is not specific and diagnosis requires a request for specific laboratory tests, diagnosis may be delayed. Delayed recognition of cases, and a 2-week incubation period add to the difficulty in attributing infections to a specific food source. From 1996-1998, an annually recurring series of outbreaks due to contaminated Guatemalan raspberries involved the USA and Canada [8]. The Cyclospora outbreak in 2013 in the USA was among the largest foodborne Illness outbreaks of 2013. The outbreak was due to contaminated salad mix (iceberg and romaine lettuce, red cabbage, and shredded carrots) and cilantro, with 631 sick people. This particular outbreak was also one of the most confusing, as at the end it appeared to be two separate Cyclospora outbreaks working in tandem. One group of illnesses was tentatively traced to a lettuce supplier in Mexico, while a second group of illnesses was linked to fresh cilantro grown in Puebla, Mexico. Because of the potential for recurrent Cyclospora outbreaks from the same source, rapidly identifying the outbreak source is critical to establishing effective control measures at the production stage.

1.3   Previous Models

Source detection models have been mostly developed in the literature of epidemiology and cybersecurity [9–11]. However, these models are non-physical Bayesian models that have never really been proven useful. [12] developed a source detection maximum likelihood estimate, which assumes virus spread in a general graph along a breadth-first-search tree and derive theoretical thresholds for the detection probability. [13] extended this estimate for partially observed transmission trees. Alternative origin reconstruction methods are based on shortest paths or spectral techniques [14] to identify a set of origin nodes on a transmission network with the knowledge of the whole outbreal time series. The limited application of these models is related to the fact that they do not include any physical factor or process in their dynamics, they have been focused on outbreak-food-pathogen attribution rather than detection of outbreak sources [15, 16], and/or they require a comprehensive knowledge of the transmission network, which is rarely the case. Moreover, these models require the whole outbreak times series which make them useless for rapid detection and response. Thus, these models have never been used in system surveillance and design. Our model is a physical-/network-based model [11, 16–19], based on the idea of replacing the conventional geographic distance by a measure of effective distance derived from the underlying food trade network and outbreak spreading patterns.

1.4   Proposed Model

The model is based on the model of [20]. Our innovation is in the coupling of such a traceback model with global sensitivity and uncertainty analyses (GSUA) [21, 22] for solving attribution uncertainty related to co-occurring outbreaks and for assessing system factor importance and identifying interactions that cause outbreaks [16]. Based on the novel notion of distance, patterns that exhibit complex spatiotemporal structure in the conventional geographic perspective turn into regular, wavelike solutions. To each outbreak pattern there is a corresponding food trade sub-network that is likely to be responsible for carrying contamination. This permits the definition of effective epidemic wave fronts, propagation speeds, and the reliable estimation of epidemic arrival times, based on the knowledge of the underlying food mobility network. The method provides two key insights. First, epidemiological factors are independent from the transport parameters, and second, the dynamics are dominated by only a small percentage of transport connections. Thus, the simplification of the food supply chain into a coarser food trade network provides an effective tool to quickly identify the likely geographic origin of the outbreak. This is also verified with the assumption of human mobility - and related travel related food contaminations

- as a second order factor. The detection of the origin of complex, multiscale dynamical spreading patterns is important for four reasons: (i) to determine what has caused the outbreak, (ii) to develop timely mitigation strategies, (iii) to predict its further spread (the arrival times in remote locations and the expected prevalence), and (iv) to map critical areas for contamination of food by looking at all observed outbreaks. This complex systems science based model also aims to identify analytics that reproduce fundamental processes without the need of extensive data that are very hard to get in reality [18, 19, 23].

2   Materials and Methods

2.1   Data

The population layer is based on the high-resolution population database of the "Gridded Population of the World project of the Socio Economic Data and Applications Center (SEDAC) that estimates the population with a granularity given by a lattice of cells covering the whole planet at a resolution of 15×15 minutes of arc. At sea level one minute of arc along the equator or a meridian equals approximately one Nautical mile (1.852 km or 1.151 mi). The International Agro-Food Trade Network (IFTN) for the USA is built using data of ComTrade [24] for the worldwide linkages among countries, and data from the United State Department of Agriculture, Foreign Agricultural Service's Global Agricultural Trade System (GATS) [25] for the trade network of imported food commodities in USA. Additional data is used from the Agricultural Marketing Service [26]. The use of both datasets allows one to cross check erroneous data and to complement missing data missing. In this case study we focused only on cilantro and fresh produce. Nodes of the network represent the countries, while the directed edges indicate the food trade fluxes among countries. Data of imported and produced food that is locally consumed is obtained from FAOSTAT food balance sheets [27]. Such information is useful for calibrating the model factor that determines how many individuals consume the contaminated food. Rainfall and temperature data are derive from the USGS, Famine Early Warning Systems Network (http://earlywarning.usgs.gov/fews/).

2.2   Effective Distance and Traceback Model

The traceback model we applied and further developed is mathematically similar to a fluid dynamics model for fluid motion characterization considering wave patterns. Such problems only require the dynamic information in a small time window, e.g., one snapshot of the wave spreading pattern. The model is based on the optimal inference of epidemiological factors that better explain the spatio-temporal occurrence of foodborne outbreaks for any potential outbreak location to which different food trade paths correspond. The range of values is determined by perturbing the estimated value of model factors as a function of the data-inferred outbreak velocity and on arrival times. All potential food commodities and outbreak sources are tested considering their likelihood to satisfy the relationship between outbreak arrival times and velocity at any time step of the epidemic and for all infected communities simultaneously. For our purposes we simplify the problem by replacing the conventional geographic distance with a probabilistically motivated distance defined as "effective distance". In the context of global, trade-mediated epidemics, we aim to use the effective distance that reliably predicts disease arrival times via epidemiological dynamics. We use the definition of effective distance D_{mn} from an arbitrary reference node n to another node m in the network as the length of the shortest path from n to m, $D_{mn} = min_\Gamma \lambda(\Gamma)$, where $\lambda(\Gamma)$ is the directed length of an ordered path $\Gamma = n_1, ..., n_L$ as the sum of effective lengths along the path. The effective distance can also be formulated as a function of the most probable food trajectories that can be derived from the connectivity matrix $\mathbf{P}$; specifically $D_{mn} = 1 - log P_{mn}$. Thus, both the average effective distance and the average shortest path trees only depend on the static mobility matrix. This implies that, on a spatial scale described by the metacommunity model, the complexity of the spatio-temporal outbreak pattern is largely determined by the structure of the mobility network (in this case of food) and not by the nonlinearities or the disease-/food-specific, epidemiological rate factors of the model. By thinking outbreak dynamics as a wave propagation pattern newtons second law applies, thus the arrival time of outbreaks is defined as

$$T_a = D_e(P)/v_e(\alpha, R_0, \gamma, \epsilon). \tag{1}$$

This equation states that the effective outbreak distances De can be computed with high fidelity based on outbreak arrival times on and effective spreading speed ve, and that each factor depends on different factors of the dynamical system considered [20]. The epidemiological factors associated with the classical SIR model determine the effective speed, whereas effective distance depends only on the topological features of the static underlying network, i.e., the matrix $\mathbf{P}$. Because, T_a and v_e is known from data (that can be in real-time), it is easy to determine D_e of an outbreak considering the uncertainty in epidemiological dynamics and in the food trade network. The geographical distance can be assessed after determining the effective distance and considering all potential food trade paths. The SIR dynamics is calibrated on the range of the observed outbreak velocity based on the maximization in space and time of the observed outbreak patterns.

2.3 Most Probable Path: Hidden Geometry Linking Patterns and Processes

The simplest method to determine which food and which outbreak source is the most likely to determine the observed outbreak patterns is to test which feasible candidate source has the lowest variability in terms of mean and variance assessed from Eq. 1. Thus, for each of the potential candidate outbreak locations, the model computes the effective distance to the subset of nodes with prevalence above a certain threshold, or just simply by looking at different instantiations of the epidemic. On the basis of this set of effective distances (denoted by different outbreak sources), we compute the $\mu_e(D_e)$ and standard deviation $\sigma_e(D_e)$ of the effective distance. As shown by [20], concentricity of epidemic waves increases with a combined minimization of mean and standard deviation of the estimated effective distance. In other words, such approach minimizes the deviation from the expected relationship arrival times distance, or velocity-distance, equivalently. It is possible to visualize the dynamics of epidemic spread and concentricity of outbreak waves by plotting outbreak sources at the center of a network where all other nodes are placed around at a radial distance equal to the effective distance. Correct outbreak sources determine cohesively evolving outbreak waves from the center to the last nodes from the beginning to the end of the epidemic.

2.4 Predictive Metacommunity Model

The metacommunity model [28, 29] consists in the coupling of a classical susceptible-infected-recovered (SIR) dynamic model with a radiation model [30] of food trade dynamics that determines the interlinked changes in food trade, contaminated food, and population state for all communities considered simultaneously. This model has the purpose to define estimates of probabilities representing average and variance dynamics of foodborne outbreaks rather than exact numbers. Contamination of food occurs as a function of combinations of values of environmental triggers, namely temperature and rainfall and such dependency is considered. Assuming that the total food trade in and out of a node is proportional to a proper combination of population sizes for the communities considered (i.e., the radiation model), the metacommunity model in which the SIR dynamics is combined with the food trade dynamics can be written as

$$\delta_t j_n = \alpha s_n j_n \sigma(j_n/\epsilon) - \beta j_n + \gamma \sum_{m \neq n} P_{mn}(j_m - j_n)$$
$$\delta_t s_n = -\alpha s_n j_n \sigma(j_n/\epsilon) + \gamma \sum_{m \neq n} P_{mn}(s_m - s_n) \,, \tag{2}$$

where $s_n = S_n/N_n$, $j_n = I_n/N_n$, and $r_n = 1 s_n j_n$. A detailed derivation of such equations is provided in [20]. The mobility parameter γ is the average food trade rate, i.e., $\gamma = \Phi/\Omega$, where $\Omega = \sum_n N_n$ is the total population in the system and $\Phi = \sum_{n,m} F_{nm}$ is the total food flux. This yields numerical values in the range $\gamma = 0.0013 - 0.0178 day^1$. The matrix P with $0 \leq P_{mn} \leq 1$ quantifies the fraction of the food flux with destination m exported from node n, i.e., $P_{mn} = F_{mn}/F_n$, where $F_n = \sum_n F_{mn}$. The additional sigmoid function $\sigma(x) = x^\eta/(1 + x^\eta)$ with gain parameter $\eta \gg 0$ accounts for the local invasion threshold ϵ and fluctuation effects for $j_n < \epsilon$. Typical ϵ and η average values are $\eta = 4, 8, \infty$ and $-log_{10}\epsilon = 4, ..., 6$. The fraction of produced and imported food that is locally consumed (that can be assessed from FAOSTAT [27]) is here governed by the input factor ϵ that is the local invasion threshold dependent on how many individuals eat the contaminated food. In general, at smaller scales it is possible to assume that consumption is proportional to the size of the population of each community. Here to avoid the use of two factors, one for local consumption and another for consumption of contaminated food, we use ϵ as the only factor determining spread of contamination. This means that we just consider the portion of consumed food that is contaminated. Moreover, we consider $\epsilon = \epsilon(T, R)$ as a function of temperature and rainfall. The variability of ϵ related to environmental variability is found via model fitting using global sensitivity and uncertainty analysis considering the assigned probability distribution. Global sensitivity and uncertainty analysis (GSUA) is here used to consider uncertainty in the traceback model and to assess the relative importance and interactions of factors epidemiological and trade network factors (Section 2.3) - leading to foodborne outbreaks. Interactions of causal factors are typically neglected as well the determination of the causality of such factors. The traceback model is run multiple times according to the Sobol scheme sampling all model factors along their probability distributions estimated from data or assumed as uniform according to a maximum entropy principle.

2.5 Food Trade Network Estimation

Most contaminations occur at production sites or at the end of the supply chain due to socio-environmental factors. For this motivation and because of the unavailable information of the whole food supply chain, we simplify the supply chain with the food trade network that is a coarse representation of the supply chain. Thus, we use a physical-based and data-verified numerical approximation of the food trade with the purpose to detect the backbone of the food supply chain that explains the observed spatio-temporal patterns of outbreaks. The magnitude of a network flux (edge weight) represents the total food (that can be expressed also as the value of the annual agro-food trade expressed in current US dollars) from one country to another represented as nodes. For the food network we use a recently introduced radiation model versus the most classical gravity model [31] that underestimates long-range trades. For this model, the connection probability of the average food mobility flux (hereafter food trade) from community i to j, is

$$Q_{ij} = \frac{H_i H_j}{(H_i + H_j)(H_i + H_j + H_{ij})} , \qquad (3)$$

where H_i and H_j is the population of the source and destination community i and j, respectively, and H_{ij} is the total population within a radius centered in i excluding the source and destination populations. The radiation model has been used for approximating the food trade in USA and Mexico in place of the gravity model commonly used by USDA. The average food trade between communities is defined for any food flux incoming in USA as $\langle F_{ij} \rangle = F_i Q_{ij}$ where F_i if the food flux from node i (i.e., an exporting country when considering external fluxes in USA). Yet, food mobility patterns are defined according to a connection matrix in which food leaves a community i for a target community j with a trade rate γ.

3   Results and Discussion

3.1   Outbreak Source Detection

The outbreak source detection model is run considering all candidate sources and food commodities. The idea is to find the optimal food-network pair that reproduces the observed outbreak patterns with the highest accuracy. The SIR simulation based on the metacommunity model with food trade determined the average value of epidemiological factors for the optimal detection of outbreak sources as: $R_0 = 1.5, \beta = 0.285 day^{-1}, \gamma = 2.8 \times 10^{-3} day-1, \epsilon = 106$ (for cilantro); and $R_0 = 1.9, \beta = 0.28 day - 1, \gamma = 2.8 \times 10 - 3 day^{-1}, and \epsilon = 10^{-6}$ (for salad mix). Such epidemiological factors are the optimal factors for reproducing the observed arrival times of outbreaks in the USA. Figure 1 depicts the correlation between arrival time and effective distance and the distribution of ensemble-normalized pairs $[\mu_e(D_e), \sigma_e(D_e)]$ for salad mix and cilantro driven outbreaks in 2013. We report the plots at the first week of the epidemic at which the identification of the outbreak source is already accurate. For all instances during the epidemic, the actual outbreak location is well separated from the remaining point cloud and closest to the origin. The variance around the 1:1 line in the arrival time effective distance plots increases with the error in estimating the distance from the real outbreak source. In an effective distance space it is possible to determine the actual outbreak source by selecting the one that maximizes the concentricity outbreak waves. Such probability distribution is related to the variability of epidemiological and trade network factors considered by global sensitivity and uncertainty analyses. Previous observations have shown that supply chain length, in-degree, betweenness centrality, and the average food trade rate are strongly driving outbreaks [16]. The local invasion threshold ϵ, that is the amount of contaminated food, is a highly interacting factor to consider as well but with lower relative importance. Epidemiological factors α and β are weakly manageable and have lower importance, which means that infection and recovery rate have small effects in decreasing the risk of outbreaks. The location of the estimated outbreak sources is shown in Fig. 2 with a probability that is related to the Nash-Sutcliffe coefficient (NSC) (Tables 1,2) considering the cumulative cases as the response variable. The root mean square error (RMSE) is also evaluated for a comprehensive assessment of how the model predicts both average trend and extremes of outbreaks over space and time [32]. Other bands of lower probability are associated with other areas in which it is less likely to find the outbreak source. The other plots in Fig. 2 show the incidence and cumulative incidence curves for both outbreak sources. The average rainfall and temperature within the evidenced areas by the dashed lined can be considered as potentially causally related to the contamination of salad and cilantro with Cyclospora in Puebla and Guanajuato. Assuming that the social determinants of contamination are the same worldwide it is possible to map the risky countries for Cyclospora contamination for which the value of rainfall and temperature is the same as the Mexico outbreak sources. A potential Cyclospora suitability can be assessed with MaxEnt [33]. Such information can be useful at smaller scale for guiding surveillance toward more risky countries.

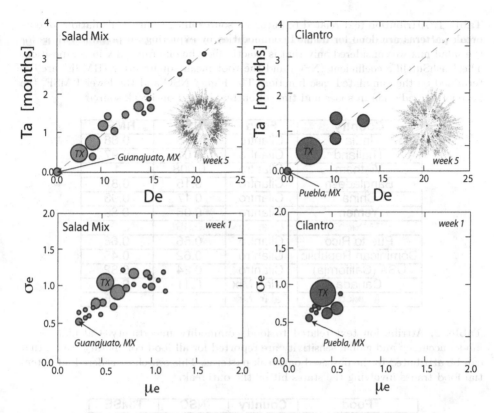

Fig. 1. Arrival time, effective distance and outbreak source detection plots. Ta is arrival time of outbreaks (from data) and De is the estimated effective distance that is related to the static trade network and the epidemiology of outbreaks in terms of arrival time of outbreak fronts. The inset shows the food trade network and the concentric expanding outbreak front in the effective distance representation. The same simulation exhibits more complex spatio-temporal patterns in the conventional geographic representation. Only the actual outbreak source produces a circular wavefront. Effective distances thus permit the extraction of the correct outbreak source, based on information on the food network and a single (or more) snapshot of the epidemic.

3.2   Detection of 2013 Outbreaks Source with Approximated Trade

The traceback model based on the effective distance is able to untangle which cases are related to cilantro and salad mix separately. This is because some outbreaks are not consistent with each other considering their co-arrival time and velocity as in Eq. 1. The highest incidence for contaminated salad mix from Guanajuato (MX) is predicted in Iowa and Nebraska, while for contaminated cilantro from Puebla (MX) is predicted in Texas (Fig. 3). The epidemiological factors are the same as the one inferred from the traceback analysis (Section 2.3). Epidemiological factors (i.e., mean infection and recovery rate) are quite invariant for the same food-pathogen pairs. Food related factors such as the mean food

Table 1. Attribution text related to outbreak source uncertainty. Calculations of outbreak patterns are done for defined commodities by exploring all possible OS; as for the salad mix we considered only that is exactly like the one from MX in composition. The NashSutcliffe coefficient (NSC) and the root mean square error (RMSE) are determined on the cumulated case function. The higher NSC and the lower RMSE, the better the prediction in space and time of outbreaks and outbreak source.

Country	Food	NSC	RMSE
India	Cilantro	0.1	0.88
Thailand	Cilantro	0.01	0.97
Vietnam	Cilantro	0.008	1
Bangladesh	Cilantro	0.15	0.87
China	Cilantro	0.17	0.93
Yemen	Cilantro	0.06	0.89
Mexico	Cilantro	0.98	0.07
Puerto Rico	Cilantro	0.56	0.66
Dominican Republic	Cilantro	0.62	0.45
USA (California)	Cilantro	0.24	0.82
Canada	Salad Mix	0.11	0.77
Mexico	Salad Mix	0.88	0.15

Table 2. Attribution text related to food commodity uncertainty. Calculations of model accuracy and global sensitivity are reported for all food commodity trades that can be attributed to the observed outbreak patterns. This search considered all potential food trades involving the states hit by the outbreak.

Food	Country	NSC	RMSE
Cantaloups	Mexico	0.31	0.714
Tomato	Mexico	0.77	0.35
Pepper Jalapeno	Mexico	0.43	0.66
Raspberries	Mexico	0.58	0.4
Raspberries	Guatemala	0.27	0.78
Cilantro	Mexico	0.98	0.07
Salad Mix	Mexico	0.88	0.15

trade, vary more but the balance of food supply and demand via trade paths has is generally very stable. Figure 4 shows how well the model predicts the observed outbreak considering one and multiple states together. Table 2 shows how the observed outbreaks can be attributed to other food commodities if the information of outbreak is not reported accurately. In the case of cilantro and fresh salad the overlap of co-contaminated cases was very high but only in the space dimension. Considering time, the spreading of salad-related outbreaks was fasted than cilantro-related outbreaks and this is an advantage that decreases the attribution ambiguity. The number of overlapping cases in 2013 were 11 at the end of the epidemic (Texas, Kansas, Nebraska, Iowa, Minnesota, Wisconsin, Illinois, Ohio, Georgia, New Jersey, and Pennsylvania). We emphasize that despite such overlap of outbreaks the proposed algorithm is able to detect the OSs after a week from the onset (Fig. 1). Moreover, we underline that the model is

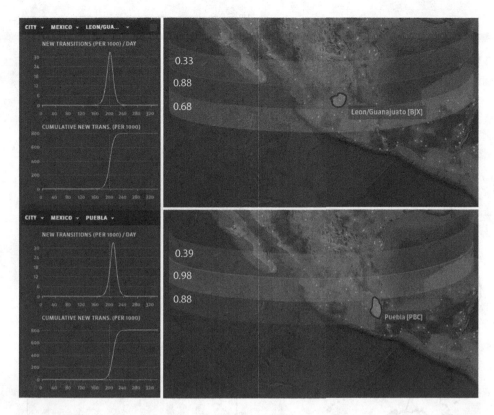

Fig. 2. Outbreak source location as main traceback model output. Outbreak sources are shown on the right at the minimum resolution of the model. Probability bands are associated to the effective distance calculations. Such probability is related to NSC and RMSE of model accuracy and prediction variability. The resolution of simulations is of 15 ? 15 minutes of arc (Section 2.1). The predicted number of cases is upscaled to the state scale to produce maps in Fig. 4.

able to disentangle cases related to different food commodities from the overall outbreak. As a matter of fact, in the summer of 2013 there was a quite extended debate whether the observed Cyclospora outbreaks were related to one of more food commodities. We believe that the availability of our traceback model would have been helpful in that and equivalent circumstances.

3.3   Prediction of 2013 Outbreaks with Unknown Source and Approximated Trade

A relevant question arises in the hypothetical case of complete uncertainty about outbreak sources. What would be the predicted outbreak pattern without the knowledge of the outbreak source? This may be the case of unsolved outbreaks or predicted outbreaks with the aim of prevention. In this study we also want to show how outbreaks patterns look like in the case of all potential sources of contaminated cilantro and salad mix are considered. Thus, we considered any

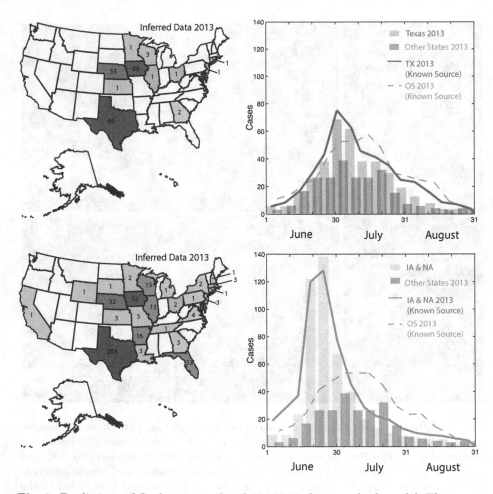

Fig. 3. Predictions of Cyclospora outbreaks in 2013 after traceback model. The trace-back model detects outbreak sources and by doing so it separates patterns of Cyclospora outbreaks due to cilantro and fresh salad contamination. Outbreaks that are not part of one epidemic wave are part of the other considering the variance-mean minimization criteria of the effective distance. The Nash-Sutcliffe coefficient and the RMSE are listed in Tables 1 and 2.

potential source of cilantro and fresh salad worldwide in which contamination occurs for the same values of environmental features in Mexico generating the 2013 outbreaks. Cilantro is grown commercially, either at small or large scale, in almost every country in the world, but most of the production is consumed in the local markets. We consider cilantro herb imported from India, Thailand, Vietnam, Bangladesh, China, Yemen, most of Latin America and the Caribbean, and from Mediterranean countries. Mexico is the largest cilantro exporter in the world, producing 42 million kg of cilantro in 5250 ha, with a farm gate value of approximately USD 13.3 million. Puerto Rico, the Dominican Republic, and

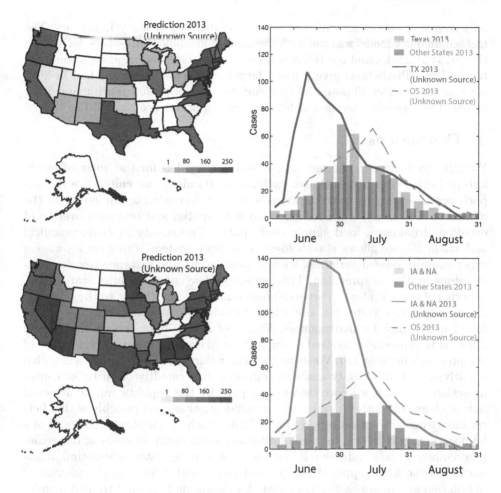

Fig. 4. Prediction of Cyclospora outbreaks in 2013 with unknow outbreak source. All the possible Oss listed in Table 1 are considered to contribute to the outbreak. Patterns of Cyclospora outbreaks due to cilantro and fresh salad contamination are more extended than the ones observed because these simulations consider all trades contaminated; thus, not only those from Mexico.

California are the other largest producers in the Americas. As for salad mix Canada and Mexico have been the leading sources of lettuce entering the United States. The two countries traded positions as the top country exporting to the United States; however, in 2002 Mexico became the leading supplier. Much of this increase in imports from Mexico is a consequence of increased romaine and leaf lettuce imports. In 2010 the United States imported 146,818 MT of all types of lettuce valued at USD 134,688 million, with more romaine and leaf lettuce being imported than head lettuce [25] Figure 4 reports the predicted outbreak patterns as if all salad and cilantro exporting countries are responsible of the outbreak. These countries are listed in Table 1 considering them separately as the only source of outbreaks with the relative prediction efficiency indicators. The metacommunity model was run with the same epidemiological factors derived fro the 2013 outbreaks, and the IFTN is used to propagate food from such countries to the USA. Predictions give a much larger spread of outbreaks than in 2013 because we consider all potential food commodity trades that reach many other states. These predictions show a 40% increase in prevalence than 2013.

4   Conclusions

We strongly believe in the use of process-based models for the quest of mechanisms behind observed outbreak patterns. Particularly, we emphasize the importance of leveraging uncertainty as a way to decrease the ambiguity in the detection of close outbreak sources even with spatial and temporal overlap of events and unknown food supply chain paths. Uncertainty in epidemiological and trade factors allows stakeholders to explore system states by leveraging other causally related variables, such as population, and distance-velocity relationships in disease spreading. Thus, models allow one to identify states (e.g., in terms of trade leading to observed outbreak patterns) closest to the observed reality and future states via alteration of trades, for instance. This has a profound importance for management. Values of model input factors that better allow us to reproduce observed outbreaks are likely the closest to real values of the processes investigated. We show that the reduction in uncertainty via global sensitivity and uncertainty analyses translates into rapidity of outbreak source detection. However, we note that in real practice this rapidity can be achieved only with an efficiently coordinated surveillance system and possibly with a better knowledge of the food supply chain. Thus, firstly we emphasize the need of a homogeneously reliable source of information about outbreak cases at fine scales (e.g. county scales) and secondly the need of a more systemic real-time information of the food supply chain for food safety and defense in the interest of population and industry. Further efforts for capturing long food trade dynamics will couple epidemiological and dynamic food supply-demand balance models driven by social and environmental triggers that determine seasonal trade, consumption, and contamination events. The potential evaluation of different design alternative of the food system as a function of climate change and land use shifts is a relevant topic also in consideration of food safety and defense. Our demonstration of this model in the context of a multistate outbreak of Cyclopsora infections associated with contaminated fresh produce highlights the potential usefulness of the model to improve the timeliness and effectiveness of outbreak detection and response. Our specific prediction strongly emphasizes the need for real-time surveillance to identify and respond to this pending outbreak.

Acknowledgments. M. Convertino acknowledges funding form the MnDRIVE Global Food Initiative at the University of Minnesota. The National Center for Food Protection and Defense (Dr. A. Kirchner in particular) is kindly acknowledged for the useful feedbacks about the paper. Funding from the Institute on the Environment at the University of Minnesota are also acknowledged.

References

1. Hoorfar, J., Jordan, K., Butler, F., Prugger, R.: Food Chain Integrity: A Holistic Approach to Food Traceability, Quality and Authenticity. Woodhead Publishing (2011)
2. Morse, S.S., Mazet, J.A.K., Woolhouse, M., et al. Prediction and prevention of the next pandemic zoonosis. Lancet (2012)
3. Kennedy, S.: Emerging global food system risks and potential solutions. In: Improving Import Food Safety. John Wiley & Sons, Inc., Hoboken (2012)
4. Kennedy, S., Busta, F.: Biosecurity: Food protection and defense. Food Microbiology: Fundamentals and Frontiers 10 (2013)
5. Meyer, S.D., Smith, K.E., Hedberg, C.: Surveillance for foodborne diseases PART 2: Investigation of foodborne disease outbreaks. In: Mikanatha, N.M., Lynfield, R., Van Beneden, C.A., et al. (eds.) Infectious Disease Surveillance (2013)
6. CDC: CDC Cyclospora investigation (2013)
7. Sanchez-Vega, J.C.F., Romero-Olmedo, H., Ortiz-Frias, A., Sokolina, J., Barreto, F.G.: Case Report: Cyclospora cayetanensis: This Emerging Protozoan Pathogen in Mexico. American Journal of Tropical Medicine and Hygiene 90(2), 351–353 (2014)
8. Ho, A.Y., Lopez, A.S., Eberhart, M.G., Levenson, R., Finkel, B.S.: Outbreak of cyclosporiasis associated with imported raspberries. Emerg. Infect. Dis. 8 (2000)
9. Gong, Y., Long, T.: Application of bayesian network in the traceback of cyber attack. In: 2010 International Conference on Computational Intelligence and Software Engineering (CiSE), pp. 1–3 (2010)
10. Xiang, Y., Li, K., Zhou, W.: Low-rate DDoS attacks detection and traceback by using new information metrics. IEEE Transactions on Information Forensics and Security 6, 426 (2011)
11. Bui-Klimke, T.R., Guclu, H., Kensler, T.W., Yuan, J.-M., Wu, F.: Aflatoxin regulations and global pistachio trade: Insights from a social network analysis. PLoS One (2014)
12. Shah, D., Zaman, T.: Detecting sources of computer viruses in networks: theory and experiment. In: Proceedings of the ACM SIGMETRICS 2010, vol. 201, pp. 203–214 (2012)
13. Pinto, P.C., Thiran, P., Vetterli, M.: Locating the source of diffusion in large-scale networks. Phys. Rev. Lett. (2012)
14. Fioriti, V., Chinnici, M.: Predicting the sources of an outbreak with a spectral technique. CoRR abs/1211.2333 (2012)
15. Wu, F., Guclu, H.: Global maize trade and food security: Implications from a social network model. Risk Analysis 33, 2168–2178 (2013)
16. Convertino, M., Liang, S.: Probabilistic supply chain risk model for food safety. GRF Davos Planet@Risk 2 (2014)
17. W.D.B.: The GLEaMviz computational tool a publicly available software to explore realistic epidemic spreading scenarios at the global scale. BMC Infect. Dis. 11, 37 (2011)
18. Vespignani, A.: Modeling dynamical processes in complex socio-technical systems. Nature Physics (2012)
19. Helbing, D., Brockmann, D., Chadefaux, T., Donnay, K., Blanke, U., Woolley-Meza, O., Moussaid, M., Johansson, A., Krause, J., Schutte, S., Perc, M.: How to Save Human Lives with Complexity Science (2014)

20. D.B.D.H.: The hidden geometry of complex network-driven contagion phenomena. Science 342, 1337–1342 (2013)
21. Saltelli, A., Ratto, M., Andres, T., Campolongo, F., Cariboni, J., Gatelli, D., Saisana, M., Tarantola, S.: Global Sensitivity Analysis (2008)
22. Convertino, M., Munoz-Carpena, R., Chu-Agor, M., Kiker, G., Linkov, I.: Untangling model drivers of species distribution predictions: Global Sensitivity and Uncertainty Analysis of MaxEnt. Env. Model & Software (2013)
23. D.L.: The parable of google flu: traps in big data analysis. Science 343, 1203–1205 (2014)
24. ComTrade (2014) (date of access: February 1, 2014)
25. GATS: USDA foreign agricultural services global agricultural trade system. Technical Report, United State Department of Agriculture (2014) (date of access: February 1, 2014)
26. AMS: Agricultural Marketing Service (2000) (date of access: March 1, 2014
27. FAOSTAT: Food balance sheet website of the food and agriculture organization of the united nations (2014) (date of access: February 2014)
28. Convertino, M., Muneepeerakul, R., Azaele, S., Bertuzzo, E., Rinaldo, A., Rodriguez-Iturbe, I.: On neutral metacommunity patterns of river basins at different scales of aggregation. Water Res. Res. (2009)
29. M.C.: Neutral metacommunity clustering and SAR: River basin vs 2-D landscape biodiversity patterns. Ecological Modeling 222 (2011)
30. F.S.: AMM, G., AL, B.: A universal model for mobility and migration patterns. Nature (2012)
31. G.P.H.R.E.I.S.L.A.: Capturing zero-trade values in gravity equations of trade: an analysis of protectionism in agro-food sectors, 141–159 (2013)
32. A.R.: R, M.C.: Performance evaluation of hydrological models: Statistical significance for reducing subjectivity in goodness-of-fit assessments (2012)
33. Anderson, S.P., Schapire, R., Maximum, R.: entropy modeling of species geographic distributions. Ecological Modelling 10 (2005)

A Case Study in Healthcare Informatics: A Telemedicine Framework for Automated Parkinson's Disease Symptom Assessment

Taha Khan[1], Mevludin Memedi[1,*], William W. Song[2], and Jerker Westin[1]

[1] Microdata Analysis Lab, Computer Engineering, Dalarna University, Borlänge, Sweden
{tkh,mmi,jwe}@du.se
[2] Microdata Analysis Lab, Informatics, Dalarna University, Borlänge, Sweden
wso@du.se

Abstract. This paper reports the development and evaluation of a mobile-based telemedicine framework for enabling remote monitoring of Parkinson's disease (PD) symptoms. The system consists of different measurement devices for remote collection, processing and presentation of symptom data of advanced PD patients. Different numerical analysis techniques were applied on the raw symptom data to extract clinically symptom information which in turn were then used in a machine learning process to be mapped to the standard clinician-based measures. The methods for quantitative and automatic assessment of symptoms were then evaluated for their clinimetric properties such as validity, reliability and sensitivity to change. Results from several studies indicate that the methods had good metrics suggesting that they are appropriate to quantitatively and objectively assess the severity of motor impairments of PD patients.

Keywords: patient monitoring, Parkinson's disease, sensors, machine learning, healthcare informatics, artificial intelligence.

1 Introduction

Healthcare Informatics (e-health) has gradually become a keen interdisciplinary research field, aiming at integration of the research fields of medicine, healthcare, and information systems and at applying modern information and telecommunication technologies in the healthcare sector [1]. There are major research activities covered in this topic including i) synthetic information analysis for medical diagnosis - collecting, analyzing and screening data from various sources, ii) healthcare information management - storing, sorting and managing patients' records and history for sharing, and iii) pervasive patients' activity monitoring. These features of e-health have been well considered in our recent studies in the case of automatic Parkinson's disease (PD) symptom analysis. This case study aims at developing and evaluating a mobile-based telemedicine framework for quantitative assessment and remote

---

* Corresponding author.

X. Zheng et al. (Eds.): ICSH 2014, LNCS 8549, pp. 197–199, 2014.
© Springer International Publishing Switzerland 2014

monitoring of PD symptoms. PD is a progressive neurological movement disorder associated with a variety of motor and non-motor symptoms. In a clinical setting today, the state of the art is to use clinical rating scales such as the Unified Parkinson's Disease Rating Scale (UPDRS) and the 39-item PD Questionnaire (PDQ-39). However, the use of these scales in clinical practice is accompanied with a number of limitations including large within- and between-clinician variability in ratings, low resolution assessments, and the need for a clinician's presence, just to name a few.

2   Methods

We have developed a telemedicine framework for remote collection, processing and presentation of symptom data of advanced PD patients. The system consists of different measurement devices including a touch screen test battery [2] with a built-in microphone [3] and a web-camera [4]. On test occasions, patients were asked to perform a set of tests including answering disease-related questions, performing fine motor tests (tapping and tracing spirals on the screen), motor speech tests by reciting standard phonetic paragraphs that were displayed on the screen, and other gross and fine motor tests such as gait and rapid finger tapping, respectively. The symptom data were then wirelessly transmitted to a central server for storage and off-line processing. Different techniques including digital signal processing, time series analysis, speech and image processing were applied on the raw symptom data to extract clinically meaningful symptom information which in turn were then used in a machine learning process to be mapped to the standard clinician-based measures like UPDRS and PDQ-39. Finally, automated scores of symptom severity were analyzed for their clinimetric properties like validity, reliability and sensitivity to treatment changes.

3   Results

The method for scoring the drawing impairment in spirals correlated well with the visual ratings of spirals given by two neurologists with a coefficient of 0.89 (P<0.001) [5]. The method for automatic assessment of alternating tapping performance of patients had good validity, test-retest reliability, sensitivity to change and ability to discriminate between patients in different disease stages and healthy elderly subjects [6]. Both these methods were also able to discriminate between different therapy-related motor states among patients [7]. In another study, an overall test score was defined by combining self-assessments and objective measures of fine motor performance in order to reflect the global health condition of the patients over week-long test periods [8]. The score had good validity when assessed against UPDRS and PDQ-39 scales with a correlation coefficient of 0.59 (P<0.001) and also was sensitive to treatment changes and could reflect the natural PD progression over time in advanced Swedish patients [9, 10]. In case of speech, features based on cepstral analysis showed strong correlation with the clinical ratings of the severity of speech symptoms with a coefficient of 0.78 (P<0.001) [3]. These features, along with some other acoustic features representing deficits in speech subsystems could classify the UPDRS levels of speech symptom severity with an accuracy of 85% [11]. In case of finger tapping, the selected features representing symptoms in the UPDRS 'Finger Tapping' item could classify between the UPDRS levels of symptom severity with an accuracy of 88% [4].

4   Conclusions

The clinical management of PD may be enhanced by application of IT-based systems composed of high-quality data collection schemes, valid and reliable data processing methods, and user-friendly graphical user interfaces. Methods for automating the process of scoring the severity of symptoms provide means for deriving precise, accurate and objective measures which can be used as outcome measures in clinical trials, enabling remote and frequent assessments. This work, through a concrete case analysis, provides a view of how these different e-health activities – diagnosis, health data management, and patient activity monitoring – will bring a great potential to healthcare and individualized medicine.

References

1. Raghupathi, W., Raghupathi, V.: Big data analytics in healthcare: promise and potential. Health. Inf. Sci. Syst. 2 (2014)
2. Westin, J., Dougherty, M., Nyholm, D., Groth, T.: A home environment test battery for status assessment in patients with advanced Parkinson's disease. Comput. Meth. Prog. Bio. 98, 27–35 (2010)
3. Khan, T., Westin, J., Dougherty, M.: Cepstral separation difference: a novel approach for speech assessment quantification in Parkinson's disease. Biocybernetics and Biomedical Engineering 34, 25–34 (2013)
4. Khan, T., Nyholm, D., Westin, J., Dougherty, M.: A computer vision framework for finger-tapping evaluation in Parkinson's disease. Artif. Intell. Med. 60, 27–40 (2014)
5. Westin, J., Ghiamati, S., Memedi, M., Nyholm, D., Johansson, A., Dougherty, M., Groth, T.: A new computer method for assessing drawing impairment in Parkinson's disease. J. Neurosci. Methods 190, 143–148 (2010)
6. Memedi, M., Khan, T., Grenholm, P., Nyholm, D., Westin, J.: Automatic and objective assessment of alternating tapping performance in Parkinson's disease. Sensors 13, 16965–16984 (2013)
7. Memedi, M., Westin, J., Nyholm, D.: Spiral drawing during self-rated dyskinesia is more impaired than during self-rated off. Parkinsonism Relat. Disord. 19, 553–556 (2013)
8. Memedi, M., Westin, J., Nyholm, D., Dougherty, M., Groth, T.: A web application for follow-up of results from a mobile device test battery for Parkinson's disease patients. Comput. Meth. Prog. Bio. 104, 219–226 (2011)
9. Westin, J., Schiavella, M., Memedi, M., Nyholm, D., Dougherty, M., Antonini, A.: Validation of a home environment test battery for supporting assessments in advanced Parkinson's disease. Neurol. Sci. 33, 831–838 (2012)
10. Memedi, M., Nyholm, D., Johansson, A., Pålhagen, S., Willows, T., Widner, H., Linder, J., Westin, J.: Self-reported symptoms and motor tests via telemetry in a 36-month levodopa-carbidopa intestinal gel infusion trial. Mov. Disord. 28, S168 (2013)
11. Khan, T., Westin, J., Dougherty, M.: Classification of speech intelligibility in Parkinson's disease. Biocybernetics and Biomedical Engineering 34, 35–45 (2014)

A Prototype Mobile Virtual Assistant for Semantic-Based Vaccine Information Retrieval

Muhammad Amith and Cui Tao*

School of Biomedical Informatics, University of Texas Health Science Center,
Houston TX 77030, USA
cui.tao@uth.tmc.edu

Abstract. Since the early 90s, healthcare providers have been mandated to provide VIS (Vaccine Information Statement) from the Centers for Disease Control and Prevention (CDC) to parents and patients before their children or themselves receive any vaccination uptake. Despite the initiative, there exist issues of patients not receiving a comprehensive understanding about the vaccines and some evidence of doubt of the safety of vaccines. In addition, a significant number of patients find vaccine information on the Internet, which may inevitably influence perceptions of vaccines. This paper introduces Vaccine Helmsman, an initial prototype of a mobile client that allows for natural language querying of semantically-driven knowledge-base of vaccine information for patients. With the ubiquitous impact of the web and mobile devices in the hands of many patients, this would allow for contextual and instant access to vaccine information, and therefore enhance vaccine literacy.

Keywords: semantic knowledge, vaccine, mHealth, ontology, natural language, mobile.

1 Vaccine Background

In the United States, the National Vaccine Childhood Injury Act mandates that all vaccine providers must distribute a Vaccine Information Statement (VIS) to the patient before any vaccine uptake [1]. VIS is *a document, produced by the CDC, that informs vaccine recipients - or their parents or legal representatives - about the benefits and risks of a vaccine they are receiving.* [1] However, studies have indicated that these documents are neglected or rarely understood by the patient or parent due to length, irrespective of the patient's social economic level [2][3]. Besides these federal documents for vaccine information, other Internet and media sources, other than the official CDC web site, has also been another source of either true and false vaccine knowledge. Several independent studies cite significant parent population that are apprehensive of vaccine uptake. Part of the reason is the success of anti-vaccination campaigns found on the Internet [4][5], increasing parental and patient fears of vaccines [6].

---

* Corresponding author.

X. Zheng et al. (Eds.): ICSH 2014, LNCS 8549, pp. 200–205, 2014.

2   Semantic Knowledge and Ontology

While the Internet allowed for the propagation of information, most information found is not uniformly consistent across various sites. These issues encourage the development and research of Semantic Web, which aims to federate a collection of data on the Internet using consistent definition of terms to express meaning and understanding, while also serializing knowledge for machines to understand. Over the last decade, efforts have been made to conceptualize vaccine knowledge to harness machine-based reasoning, integration with other knowledge bases and domains, and standardizing vaccine knowledge [7]. The HeGroup research team from University of Michigan has done substantial work in the development of knowledge bases and tools for ontology-based vaccines [8] and adverse effects of vaccines [9]. However, the vaccine and adverse effects of vaccine ontologies are directed for medical professionals familiar with the knowledge domain's lexicon, and may not be suitable for the general population to understand.

3   Ontology-Driven Mobile Applications and Natural Language Interfaces

The last few years, the web traffic originating from mobile devices have exponentially grown, and the accessibility of mobile devices in the hands of most of the of the world population make it a natural candidate to deliver vaccine information. Recently, there has been no shortage of studies for utilization of mobile devices and semantic knowledge, especially in healthcare. Lakehead University developers introduced MORF (Mobile Health Monitoring Platform), which monitors a patient's health status through a Bluetooth sensor and relays the vitals to a Nokia phone [10] [11]. The device then sends the data to a knowledge management server, making system decisions based on the ontological model and the Jess expert rule-based framework. A similar system also follows the same idea of patient monitoring with an Android prototype that monitors diabetic patients [12].

Along with ontology-driven mobile smartphones, there has been growing incorporation of voice enabled user interaction with commercial software [13] using natural language interfaces (NLI). NLI *is a system that allows users to access information stored in some repository by formulating the request in natural language* [14]. These applications fall between either handling constrained vocabulary (pre-defined accepted commands) or unconstrained vocabulary (no limit on words or phrases accepted), and tend to employ a thick client or thin client architecture, where the speech handling occurs on the server [15]. Some well-known implementations are Apple's Siri [16], Android's Now [17], or Samsung's S Voice [18], which facilitates basic mobile device functions through speech commands. Review of the current literature have revealed more domain-specific use cases, like VAMATA prototype, following the same concept as intelligent personal assistant but utilizes a knowledge base for medical military domain [19].

However, the precision of natural language interfaces is dependent on the domain to avoid any ambiguity in speech [20] [14]. Despite this limitation, there is research interest in making NLI portable and independent of certain domains.

4   Vaccine Helmsman - A Prototype Mobile Virtual Assistant for Semantic-Based Vaccine Information Retrieval

Culling lessons from the above-mentioned examples, the authors proposes the utilization of mobile devices and natural language interfaces to retrieve vaccine knowledge represented in a semantic knowledge system - Vaccine Helmsman.

4.1   VISO - Vaccine Information Statement Ontology

The main driver for this mobile project is the utilization of semantic knowledge bases that permit the development of a natural language interface for patients and parents to utilize voice commands to query vaccine knowledge. We are developing the Vaccine Information Statement Ontology (VISO) for semantically representing vaccine knowledge in consumer vocabulary for this purpose. The VISO ontology is represented in the Web Ontology Language (OWL) [21], which is a standard ontology language for the Semantic Web community. For this prototype, the project models two vaccines - Hepatitis B and Rotavirus. Later progression of this project will refine the knowledge model to accommodate additional vaccine information from CDC vaccine statements. The project utilizes Protégé 4.3 [22] to develop and serialize the knowledge base of both Hepatitis B and Rotavirus.

4.2   System Architecture

In conjunction with the creation of VISO ontology, the authors have developed a prototype iOS application in Objective-C that feed in voice commands and process the command to retrieve a response from a remote web server (See Figure 1). Two major decomposition of the Vaccine Helmsman application - a natural language interface (NLI) and command-to-query translator - have been developed. The function of the NLI will be major front-end component that will coordinate the speech interaction between the user and the system. It will also be responsible for validating the commands and sending commands to the translator. The translator's component will align the speech command to an appropriate query request, which will then be sent to a remote server in JSON [23]. Once data is received from the server, the application constructs a semi-structured speech response to answer the user request. At the current stage, the prototype is limited to only pre-defined template commands to suggest possible vaccine retrieval option. Later research goals will involve more flexible speech commands and responses to be discussed in the future direction section.

Also deployed is the Jena Fuseki [24] application component that will retrieve the command from the application and query for a response to be sent back to the device - in speech and text. The Fuseki triplestore server will host the serialized VISO OWL file. The Vaccine Helmsman architecture is shown below in Figure 1.

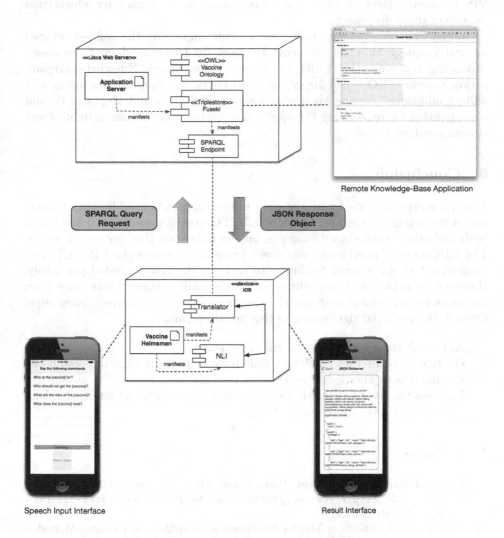

Fig. 1. Vaccine Helmsman system architecture

5 Limitations and Future Direction

Currently, the prototype implementation's offline speech recognition vocabulary is limited to approximately 300-500 words. This may or may not limit possibility to allow for more unconstrained speech commands. The authors also foresee the possibility of non-English speaking patients, particularly Spanish speakers in the US, who may benefit from vaccine knowledge. This would also imply that VISO will need to incorporate multilingual equivalent terms, as well as synonymous terms. While the VISO knowledge base is derived from the CDC's VIS documents, the authors recognize that users may need auxiliary information outside of those documents.

Subsequent development efforts will include improving the semi-structured natural language limitation to allow for more fluid commands and responses; expanding and evaluating VISO, like incorporating Simple Knowledge Organization System (SKOS) [25] for synonymous terms and multilingual terms, and adding additional vaccine knowledge beyond Rotavirus and Heptatis B; and consideration for redesigning the application design architecture in light of any system constraints.

6 Conclusion

This prototype appears to be the only unique application addressing vaccine knowledge retrieval using speech commands. There exist experimental web-based tools and other mobile-based concepts, but no indication they are mobile-ready. The CDC website provides a mobile-web template to access the VIS PDF documents, yet it is not a valid solution to some of the issues alluded previously. However, in other use cases outside of vaccine information, there have been attempts to experiment with mobile speech commands to retrieve knowledge. Overall, the potential significance of this prototype may:

- Aid in alleviating vaccine concerns of patients;
- Overcome the literacy challenges that prevent patients from understanding vaccine related knowledge; and
- Progress the use of mHealth tools that harness retrieval of knowledge-base systems and speech interfaces.

References

1. Vaccine Information Statement: Facts About VISs - Vaccines - CDC (published June 18, 2013), http://www.cdc.gov/vaccines/hcp/vis/about/facts-vis.html (accessed March 1, 2014)
2. Lieu, T., et al.: Effects of Vaccine Information Pamphlets on Parents' Attitudes. Arch. Pediatr. Adolesc. Med. 148, 921–925 (1994)
3. St-Amour, M., et al.: Are vaccination information leaflets useful for vaccinators and parents? Vaccine 24, 2491–2496 (2006)
4. Kata A. A postmodern Pandora's box: Anti-vaccination information on the Internet. Vaccine 28, 2010: 1709-1715.
5. Kata, A.: Anti-vaccine activists, Web 2.0, and the postmodern paradigm - An overview of tactics and tropes used online by the anti-vaccination movement. Vaccine 30, 3778–3789 (2012)

6. Olpinski, O.. Anti Vaccination Movement and Parental Refusals of Immunization of Children in USA. Pediatria Polska 87, 381–385 (2012)

7. He, Y.: VO: Vaccine Ontology. University of Michigan (2009)

8. VO: Vaccine Ontology, http://www.violinet.org/vaccineontology/ (accessed March 1, 2014)

9. OAE, http://www.oae-ontology.org/ (accessed March 1, 2014)

10. Docksteader, L., Benlamri, R.: Mobile Ontology-based Reasoning and Feedback (MORF) Health Monitoring System. In: Third International Conference on Digital Information Management, ICDIM, vol. 2008, pp. 876–880. IEEE (2008)

11. Docksteader, L., Benlamri, R.: MORF: A Mobile Health-Monitoring Platform. IEEE Computer Society, IT Pro, 18–25 (May/June 2010)

12. Villarreal, V., Fontescha, J., Hervas, R., Bravo, J.: Mobile and ubiquitous architecture for the medical control of chronic diseases through the use of intelligent devices: Using the architecture for patients with diabetes. Future Generation Computer Systems 34, 161–175 (2014)

13. Massie, T., Wijesekera, D.: TVIS: Tactical Voice Interaction Services for Dismounted Urban Operations. In: Military Communications Conference, MILCOM 2008, November 16-19, pp. 16–19. IEEE (2008)

14. Kaufmann, E., Bernstein, A.: Evaluating the Usability of Natural Language Query Languages and Interfaces to Semantic Web Knowledge Bases. Web Semantics: Science, Services and Agents on the World Wide Web 8(4), 377–398 (2010)

15. Kurschl, W., Mitsch, S., Prokop, R., Schonbock, J.: Development Issues for Speech-Enabled Mobile Applications. In: proceeding of: Software Engineering 2007, Fachtagung des GI-Fachbereichs Softwaretechnik, pp. 27–30 (2007)

16. Siri, A.: http://www.apple.com/ios/siri/ (accessed March 1, 2014)

17. Google Now, http://www.google.com/landing/now/ (accessed March 1, 2014)

18. Samsung S Voice, http://www.samsung.com/global/galaxys3/svoice.html (accessed March 1, 2014)

19. James, G., Roger, J.: Mobile Speech and the Armed Services: Making a Case for Adding Siri-like Features to VAMTA (Voice-Activated Medical Tracking Application). Mobile Speech and Advanced Natural Language Solution, pp. 319–323. Springer (2013)

20. Kopsa, J., Mikovec, Z., Slavik, P.: Ontology driven voice-based interaction in mobile environment. Dagstuhl Seminar. In: Proceedings 05181 Mobile Computing and Ambient Intelligence: The Challenge of Multimedia. Internationales Begegnungs- und Forschungszentrum (August 12, 2005)

21. OWL 2 Web Ontology Language Document Overview, 2nd edn., http://www.w3.org/TR/owl2-overview/ (accessed April 25, 2014)

22. Protégé, http://protege.stanford.edu/ (accessed March 10, 2014)

23. JSON, http://json.org/ (accessed April 25, 2014)

24. Fuseki.: Serving RDF data over HTTP, https://jena.apache.org (accessed April 24, 2014)

25. SKOS Simple Knowledge Organization System, http://www.w3.org/2004/02/skos/ (Accessed April 25, 2014)

Supportive Glucose Sensing Mobile Application to Improve the Accuracy of Continuous Glucose Monitors[*]

Ahmed Gomaa[1,**], Chaogui Zhang[1], Muhammad Hasan[2], Mary Beth Roche[3], and Shaun Hynes[1]

[1] Marywood University, Scranton, PA
{agomaa,czhang,shynes}@marywood.edu
[2] Texas A&M International University, Laredo, TX
muhammad.hasan@tamiu.edu
[3] Lackawanna College, Scranton, PA
rochem@lackawanna.edu

Abstract. An insulin pump can be programmed to continuously deliver accurate amounts of insulin to diabetic patients. A continuous glucose monitor (CGM) which provides continuous patient glucose levels, needs to be calibrated at least every 6 hours. This paper provides an overview of the software and hardware requirements to increase the calibration duration with a high level of accuracy in an open source Artificial Pancreas platform. On the software level, it uses a smartphone camera to capture the food intake, and a smartphone sensor and positioning system to capture the patient movements. The system maps three months' worth of data points to the actual glucose level generated by the CGM. It then generates the probability of the estimated insulin needed based on the recorded movements and food intake activities for the patient. The logged data is used as the training data set. Using Bayes' analysis, the generated probability that is based on the patient activities is used as posterior probabilities to the CGM results, which generates a more accurate estimation of the glucose level. On the hardware level, the paper presents a Universal Remote Control and its associated protocol to connect the smartphone with the CGM for information retrieval and with the insulin pump for information dissemination. The information is sent to the insulin pump using a Field Programmable Gate Array (FPGA). For communication, there are two kinds of message frames: Dosage Delivery Frame (DDF) and Acknowledgement frame (ACKF) with a secure layer of encryption.

Keywords: Continuous glucose monitor (CGM), Insulin pump, Bayes' analysis, Field Programmable Gate Array (FPGA), Diabetes.

---

[*] This work is being sponsored in part by Murray Award for Research and Development for 2013-2014 and TecBridge/Northeastern Pennsylvania Technology Institute (NPTI).
[**] Corresponding author.

X. Zheng et al. (Eds.): ICSH 2014, LNCS 8549, pp. 206–212, 2014.

1   Introduction

Diabetes is a disorder of metabolism where the body has trouble using glucose, or blood sugar, for energy. When we eat, our body breaks down foods known as carbohydrates (fruits, vegetables, breads, pastas, dairy, and sweets) into glucose, which is sent to our cells through the bloodstream as energy. Insulin is a hormone, secreted from the pancreas, that is needed to convert glucose into the energy needed for daily life [1]. The activity levels of diabetics and the amount of carbohydrate intake can help determining how much insulin is needed throughout the day [2]. Since 1974, the scientific community started to acknowledge the fact that an artificial pancreas is a possibility [3]. An Artificial Pancreas System, interchangeably called a closed-loop system includes three main components, a continuous glucose monitoring system (CGM), an insulin infusion pump, and a control algorithm [4]. A continuous glucose monitoring system (CGM) is used to calculate the appropriate insulin and glucagon infusion level to achieve the specified target of insulin blood level. [5, 6]. An insulin infusion pump is a small device that is worn externally and delivers precise doses of insulin and glucagon to closely match the body's needs. A commercial wireless device controls the pump dosage to the body. This technology has been approved by the FDA in 2012. At present, the device is controlled by a commercially available application (OmniPod® Insulin Management System). A control Algorithm and a supervisor control analyze the output from the CGM and send the required amount of infusion to the insulin infusion pump. Several methodologies of control Algorithm are used including proportional integral derivative control [7], fuzzy logic control [8], and rule based algorithms [9] to name a few.

2   Research Problem

There are a number of challenges to have a fully automated and accurate Artificial Pancreas system, including:

- The need to calibrate existing CGM every six hours to maintain accurate reading, [10] . A 2013 prototype CGM system reports an 83.4% accuracy rate, when compared to clinically accurate results [11]. The inaccurate results from CGM systems are considered one of the main obstacles of Artificial Pancreas [4].
- The acknowledged problem of the vast amount of patents granted in the close-loop / Artificial Pancreas systems domain increased from 24 patents in 1991 to 247 patents in 2001 in the United States alone. Figure 1 and Figure 2 depicts the two main strategies used to currently create a close-loop system [12]. This leads to the risk of infringement of already existing patents and diabetic patients may not have access to inexpensive closed-loop system.

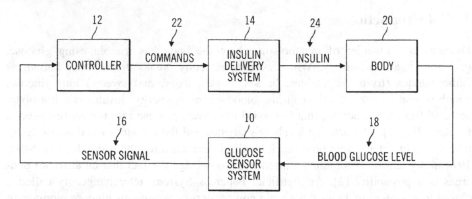

Fig. 1. Figure 1 of U.S. Patent 6,558,351 B1: proportional integral derivative (PID) controller

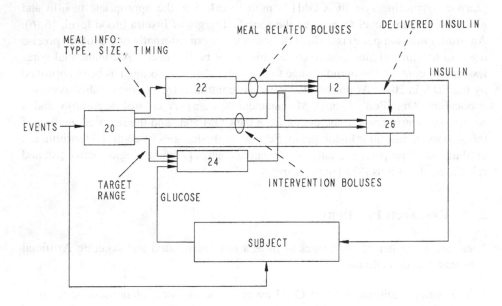

Fig. 2.   Figure 5 of U.S. Patent 6,544,212 B2: model predictive controller (MPC)

3   Methodology

To improve the accuracy of the CGM systems, we propose adding to the CGM systems output the posterior probabilities of the patients' insulin levels based on their estimated food intake and activities. We plan on using smartphones as receptacles for the monitoring activities of the patients, as well as the host of the control algorithm, where it calculates the final results, and send them to the insulin pump for infusion. To achieve this, we will need a hardware component to retrieve information from the CGM away from their typical patented communication channel, and to bypass the insulin pump current patented communication channel to infuse the insulin.

Preferably, we need a *Universal Remote Control* which will enable us to create an open source platform, to send and receive messages to and from an Artificial Pancreas System. Additionally, we use the smartphone to improve on the results of the un-calibrated CGM devices by incorporating the captured patient daily activity using the smartphone camera, Global Positioning System and motion sensors as posterior probability to the current patient level insulin need as distributed by the CGM.

4   System Architecture

4.1   Software

The mobile app will provide users with a convenient way to track their blood sugar level, food intake and physical activity, and also manage their insulin amount efficiently. In the first phase of development, all information is inserted manually, in the second phase, the Global Positioning System and motion sensors coordinates will be recorded, and in the third phase the app will include an image base retrieval system that matches the food intake captured by the phone camera and based on the food similarity, it will estimate the initial amount of carbohydrates in each meal using existing image base retrieval systems. The results during a three month period of using the system would create a trend line that can be measured against the actual level of glucose in the blood from the CGM. A comparison between different data mining models will take place to identify the most suitable predictive model that matches the captured user behavior and her actual insulin needs. The resulting coefficient from the selected model is used to estimate the level of expected insulin required. The probability of the resulting insulin required will be a posterior probability using Naïve Base analysis to identify the probability of the actual required insulin.

In the first phase of development, each user sets up a profile upon first use of the app. This includes basic information such as name, age, gender, weight, height, as well as diabetes management related information such as length of diabetes condition, doctor information, type, frequency and dosage of insulin recommended/prescribed by the doctor. The user also has the option of setting up a schedule for insulin injection, and the app can use that as an alarm/reminder for the user.

The app provides an easy to use interface for users to record their blood sugar level at each testing. The glucose level can also be plotted easily to allow the user to conveniently visualize the fluctuation pattern, and compare it with the desired/target level.

At either scheduled times or before meals/snacks, the user can enter information such as the current blood sugar level, planned food intake (amount/type), and physical activities. The app will calculate the amount of insulin based on the user input. The calculation will be dynamically adjusted based on the historical blood sugar level and the desired/intended level.

User data is securely stored on the mobile device, and the user can setup different access control modes of the app, to ensure convenience and privacy. The user also has the option of backing up the data to computers or cloud services. Doing so would secure the user data in the event of the mobile device becoming lost or stolen.

4.2   Remote Control and Insulin Pump

An insulin pump can be programmed to continuously deliver tiny and precise amounts of insulin twenty-four hours a day. This is called the basal rate and can maintain normal glucose levels between meals and continue overnight. Alternatively, it can effortlessly deliver additional insulin, called a bolus dosage, to cover the extra glucose from a meal or to correct a high blood glucose reading [13]. At this point we are considering only a bolus dosage.

To create an open platform and a universal remote control to bypass any patented communication channel, and to promote interoperability between different close-loop system components, we introduce a *Universal Remote Control*. The interface between the *Universal Remote Control* and the smart phone could use Wi-Fi technology. This interface is often available in smartphones. Interface between the remote control and the insulin pump could be Bluetooth® or unlicensed-ISM-band receivers. Some pumps have RF receivers (using these protocols) to obtain data from continuous glucose monitors [14].

The *Universal Remote Control* receives the insulin dosage information from a smart phone. Then the remote control will create an appropriate message format (with this dosage information) for the protocol to deliver the message to the insulin pump. This operation of the remote control can be achieved by using an embedded processor or a Field Programmable Gate Array (FPGA).

There should be two kinds of message frames namely Dosage Delivery Frame (DDF) and Acknowledgement frame (ACKF). In order to ensure security, the message frames should be encrypted [14]. High quality encryption such as Data Encryption Standard (DES) or better algorithm may be employed [15].

Once the insulin pump receives the DDF, it responds with ACKF to the remote control. Then it should be able to decrypt and interpret the frame in order to find out the insulin dosage information. Based on the dosage information, it should be able to find out the displacement necessary for the plunger. Then it should apply necessary signals to the motor controlling the plunger.

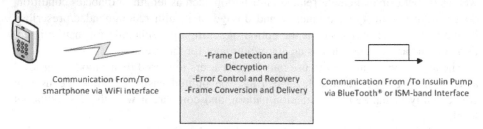

Fig. 3. Communication between Smartphone and Insulin Pump

The encoder connected to the motor shaft could ensure that the necessary rotation has occurred for the motor to displace the plunger and for the delivery of insulin from the cartridge [14]. At that point, the insulin pump should reply back to the remote control that dosage has been delivered. It needs to use a Dosage Delivery Confirmation Frame (DDCF) to convey this message. Once the insulin pump receives ACKF from the remote control, the dosage delivery session will end.

5 Discussion

In this paper we presented a framework overview to improve the accuracy of a CGM system using smartphones, by incorporating the user activities in the estimation of the required insulin, but adding the insulin requirement probability as a posterior probability to the insulin level recommended from the CGM system. This should address the requirement to recalibrate the CGM system every 6 hours. In addition, we presented an overview of a *Universal Remote Control* to enable the creation of an open platform for close-loop / Artificial Pancreas systems by adding an FPGA to the CGM and the insulin pump and using a proposed communication framework.

There are a number of challenges to achieve our overview that must be addressed to reach to this conclusion. Initially, smartphones are not ready to gain a class III high risk medical devices [4]. There are unaddressed problems including the battery life, the sensors accuracy, and the stickiness of the smartphone to the patient and the accuracy of the image retrieval system in determining the amount of carbs from the taken pictures. In addition, a safety control in terms of the device malfunction, as well as the privacy controls.

References

1. Barnett, T., Kumar, S.: Obesity and Diabetes, 2nd edn. Wiley, Hobken (2009)
2. Centers for Disease Control and Prevention (CDC), National diabetes fact sheet: National estimates and general information on diabetes and prediabetes in the United States, 2011. US Department of Health and Human Services, Centers for Disease Control and Prevention, Atlanta (2011)
3. Albisser, A., et al.: An artificial endocrine pancreas. Diabetes 23, 389–396 (1974)
4. Peyser, T.: The artificial pancreas: Current status and future prospects. Annals Of The New York Academy of Sciences 1311, 102–123 (2014)
5. Staff, The Content of Investigational Device Exemption (IDE) and Premarket Approval (PMA) Applications for Artificial Pancreas Device Systems. Guidance for Industry and Food and Drug Administration (2012)
6. O'Grady.: The use of an automated, portable glucose control system for overnight glucose control in adolescents and young adults with type 1 diabetes. Diabetes Care (2012)
7. Steil, G.: Feasibility of automating insulin delivery for the treatment of type 1 diabetes. Diabetes 55, 3344–3350 (2006)
8. Phillip, M.: Nocturnal glucose control with an artificial pancreas at a diabetes camp. N. Engl. J. Med. 368, 824–833 (2013)
9. Wang, Y.: Algorithm for the artificial pancreatic b-cell. Diabetes 12, 879–887 (2010)
10. Yue, X.-Y.: Real-Time Continuous Glucose Monitoring Shows High Accuracy within 6 Hours after Sensor. PLoS ONE 3(8) (2013)
11. Zschornack: Evaluation of the performance of a novel system for continuous glucose monitoring. J. Diabetes Sci. 7, 815–823 (2013)
12. Erdin, N.: Further Development of Artificial Pancreas: Blocked by Patents? J. Diabetes Sci. Technol. 2(6), 971–976 (2008)

13. Staff, Insulin Pump Therapy for Type 1 Diabetes,
    http://www.medtronic-diabetes.com.au (accessed March 30, 2014)
14. Staff, Insulin pumps Home Medical Application notes,
    http://www.maxim-ic.com/medical (accessed March 30, 2014)
15. Paul, T.: A Review of the Security of Insulin Pump Infusion Systems. Journal of Diabetes
    Science Technology 5(6), 1557–1562 (2011)

A Control Study on the Effects of HRV Biofeedback Therapy in Patients with Post-Stroke Depression

Xin Li[1], Tong Zhang[1], Luping Song[1], Yong Zhang[2], Chunxiao Xing[2], and Hsinchun Chen[2,3]

[1] School of Rehabilitation Medicine, Capital Medical University, Bejing, China
[2] Research Institute of Information Technology,
Tsinghua National Laboratory for Information Science and Technology,
Department of Computer Science and Technology, Tsinghua University, Beijing, China
[3] Artificial Intelligence Lab, University of Arizona
horsebackdancing@sina.com, zt61611@sohu.com,
songluping882002@aliyun.com,
{zhangyong05,xingcx}@tsinghua.edu.cn, hchen@eller.arizona.edu

Abstract. The post-stroke is often associated with emotional disorders, among which post-stroke depression (PSD) has a high incidence. We applied Heart Rate Variability (HRV) biofeedback to train PSD patients by a prospective randomized control study. The purpose of this study was to investigate the effectiveness of the HRV biofeedback on stroke patients' emotional improvement, autonomic nerve function and prognostic implications. In the feedback group, the patients had learned to breathe at the resonant frequency to increase their low frequency (LF) as well as adjust their respiration to synchronize with heart rate fluctuations. Our findings suggest that the HRV biofeedback may be a valid treatment especially on the improvement of depression levels and sleep disturbance in PSD patients.

Keywords: Heart Rate Variability, Biofeedback, Stroke, Depression.

1 Introduction

The post-stroke is often associated with emotional disorders, among which post-stroke depression (PSD) has a high incidence [1,2]. Post-stroke depression is one of the common complications of cerebrovascular diseases. It not only worsens the physical symptoms of patients, which brings physical and mental distress to them, but also seriously affects the recovery of neurological function and delays that of neurological deficit. Drug therapy and cognitive behavioral therapy are mostly used in current clinical treatment of PSD. Yet patients often have a poor response to the later, and the former has problems such as slow onset of action and various side effects. A more economic and simple intervention procedure with no adverse reactions is required. Heart rate variability (HRV) biofeedback requires patients to synchronize fluctuations in breathing and heart rate by slow abdominal breathing (about 5.5 to 6 times per minute, i.e. at the resonance frequency of 0.1Hz), and thus maximize heart

X. Zheng et al. (Eds.): ICSH 2014, LNCS 8549, pp. 213–224, 2014.
© Springer International Publishing Switzerland 2014

rate variability. From many experiments, we found that HRV biofeedback can improve HRV indexes and / or baroreflex function [3,4], scientists abroad have already had studies on using HRV biofeedback treatment on anxiety and depression, and found a significant clinical efficacy. There is evidence indicated that PSD patients have problems with HRV reduction and baroreflex function decline, which means that the patients' autonomic nervous system dysfunction has been severely damaged, and the body has poor ability to adapt to the changed physiological environment. As an important auxiliary method of standard treatments program, it has been proved that HRV biofeedback can improve the regulatory function of the autonomic nervous system, and take intervention especially on the autonomic nervous system dysfunction for PSD patients. Moreover, the most important thing is that the non-drug treatment shall definitely bring about none of side effects of drugs. Literature search found few studies on HRV biofeedback in post-stroke depression both at home and abroad. The purpose of the experiment is to study the impacts of HRV biofeedback on patients' emotional improvement, autonomic nervous function and prognosis, and the study will accumulate some precious experiences for clinical practice and promotion, and surely become a beneficial supplement for comprehensive recovery.

2   Design and Subjects

2.1   Inclusion and Exclusion Criteria

Subjects of the study were rehabilitation inpatients in Beijing Bo Ai Hospital from February 2012 to May 2013. Eligible patients met the following conditions: ①Aged 18 to 75 years old, male or female; ②Meeting the diagnostic criteria for stroke confirmed by head CT or MRI, and in first episode of stroke accompanied by limb movement disorder [5]; ③Meeting the diagnostic criteria of depression status with no psychotic symptoms developed in International Classification of Diseases (ICD-10), with or without anxiety [6], and having a total score greater than 20 according to Hamilton Depression Scale (HAMD,24-items version); ④Stable vital signs verified by the test taken in 2-6 months after stroke onset; ⑤ Conscious, of complete orientation, and with no apparent memory disorders, understanding barriers or mental retardation; ⑥Primary education and above; ⑦Able to cope with the completion of testing and treatment, and having signed informed consent. Patients were excluded for any of the following reasons: ① Depression status with psychotic symptoms; ② Previous history of mental disorders and emotional disorders; ③Associated with severe lung infections, central respiratory failure, electrolyte imbalance, fever and other diseases affecting the heart activity; ④Associated with other organic diseases, previous history of arrhythmias (atrial fibrillation and frequent premature beats), hyperthyroidism, history of syncope and autonomic nervous system dysfunction, or the application of drugs and substances affecting the activity of the autonomic nervous found by detection; ⑤ Serious consciousness disturbance, dementia, cognitive impairment and aphasia; ⑥Brainstem infarction; ⑦Severe dysarthria and dysphagia; ⑧Accidents in family or stressful life events recently(such as death of spouse, death of children and getting laid off, etc.); ⑨Unable to cooperate or comply with treatment programs , and unable to grasp the essentials of breathing after training 5 times in the feedback group.

2.2   General Conditions of Subjects

24 patients enrolled in the experiment were divided into feedback and control groups according to the Randomized Controlled Trials Table [7] under the principle of voluntary, with 13 in the feedback group and 11 in the control group. In the feedback group, patients completed the experiment were composed of 5 males and 8 females, aged 54.38±13.33 with disease course lasting 3.62±2.18 months, left/right hemiparesis=10/3, 8 patients with cerebral infarction, 5 with cerebral hemorrhage and all in first onset except one who had relapsed cerebrovascular disease (over 1 year after last onset and no squeal like lacunar infarction). All patients had signed informed consent.

2.3   Grouping

All the 24 patients were given conventional rehabilitation including exercise therapy, occupational therapy, physical therapy, traditional Chinese medicine, psychotherapy and medication. The feedback patients were given additional heart rate variability biofeedback therapy (30 minutes a time, 3 times a week for 4-6 weeks, and 10 times as a course). While the control patients were tested by the computer software to carry out the treatment relaxation therapy without a feedback signal to make them breathe quietly and stay awake. The effects were evaluated by Hamilton Depression Scale (HAMD), Hamilton Anxiety Scale (HAMA), Pittsburgh Sleep Quality Index (PSQI), the simplified Fugl-Meyer motor Assessment (FMA), the National Institutes of Health Stroke Scale (NIHSS), the Modified Barthel Index (MBI) and the monitoring of each physiological parameter (EMG, skin temperature, galvanic skin response, heart rate variability, etc.) produced by Multi-channel biofeedback instrument before and after treatment respectively.

2.4   Equipments and Materials

HRV biofeedback training was conducted in the biofeedback and cognitive laboratory of Beijing Bo Ai Hospital. The temperature was maintained at 24 - 26 °C, and the humidity was kept between 60% with 70%. The room should be kept quiet and with no significant air flow. Electronic devices except the biofeedback equipments should be shut down before conducting the treatment, and outside interference should be avoided in the process. Equipments for biofeedback training were VBFB type biofeedback system, named VBFB-3000 (dual display) and provided by Nanjing Vishee Medical Technology Co., Ltd. The software system used was the Chinese version of BioNeuro Infiniti 5.1. It conducted 3 minutes' short-term time- and frequency-domain analysis on the HRV data collected. Indices of HRV time-domain analysis included standard deviation of normal RR intervals (SDNN) and heart rate

(HR), and indices of frequency-domain analysis included low frequency LF, high frequency HF and LF / HF ratio. To get a normal distribution of data collected, we used Fast Fourier transform (FFT) option for logarithmic conversion of indices of HRV frequency domain analysis.

2.5   Statistical Analysis

We evaluated the differences between the two groups. Paired samples t-tests on data before and after the experiment and one-way analysis of variance on data of the two groups were calculated with the application of SPSS software package. When the data is not normally distributed, the Wilcoxon rank-sum non-parametric tests were used to compare the data before and after the experiment and between two groups.

3   Results

3.1   Impacts of HRV Biofeedback on Emotion

Impacts on Depression. There were significant differences in the following factors in the feedback group before and after treatment, that was, Anxiety/Somatization factor score (from 6.18 ± 2.40 to 2.55 ± 1.70, P=0.00), Cognitive impairment factor score (from 3.27 ± 1.95 to 0.82 ± 1.25, P=0.00), Total Score of HAMD (from 25.73 ± 5.36 to 11.45 ± 5.56, P=0.00), Weight factor score (from 0.91 ± 0.70 to 0.18 ± 0.41, P=0.02), Block factor score (from 6.27 ± 1.49 to 2.55 ± 1.81, P=0.01) and Desperation factor score (from 4.64 ± 1.69 to 2.64 ± 1.03, P=0.02) in HAMD scale. Scores of the above factors all decreased after treatment. While in the control group, only Anxiety/Somatization factor score (from 5.13 ± 1.81 to 3.13 ± 2.03, P=0.05) had a significant difference, also with score decreasing, as shown in Table 1 and Table 2.

Table 1. Comparison of HAMD Factors and Total Score ($\bar{x} \pm s$, t)

Item	Group	Baseline	F	Sig.	Follow-up	F	Sig.
Anxiety/ Somatization	Feedback Group (n=13)	6.18±2.40	1.09	0.31	2.55±1.70[&&] && P=0.00	0.46	0.51
	Control Group (n=11)	5.13±1.81			3.13±2.03[&] & P=0.05		
Cognition impairment	Feedback Group (n=13)	3.27±1.95	0.01	0.92	0.82±1.25[&&] && P=0.00	1.14	0.30
	Control Group (n=11)	3.38±2.33			1.38±0.92		
Sleep disturbance	Feedback Group (n=13)	3.55±2.42	1.67	0.21	1.91±2.07	7.88	0.01*
	Control Group (n=11)	4.88±1.89			4.38±1.60		
Total Scores	Feedback Group (n=13)	25.73±5.36	0.45	0.51	11.45±5.56[&&] && P=0.00	4.23	0.06
	Control Group (n=11)	23.63±8.28			16.88±5.84		

Note: [&] Comparison of the feedback group before and after treatment P<0.05, [&&] Comparison of the feedback group before and after treatment P<0.01, *Comparison of the two groups P<0.05, ** Comparison of the two groups P<0.01. The Notes in following Tables are the same with this Note.

Sleep disturbance factor score (F=7.88, P=0.01) and Block factor score (Z=-2.10, P=0.04) showed significant differences after treatment, of which the scores in the feedback group were apparently lower than those of the control group. The Total Score of feedback group was lower, with the value of P close to 0.05(F=4.32, P=0.06), as shown in Table 1 and Table 2.

Table 2. Comparison of HAMD Factors and Total Score ($\overline{x} \pm s$, sum of ranks)

Item	Group	Baseline	Z	Sig.	Follow-up	Z	Sig.
Weight	Feedback Group（n=13）	0.91±0.70	-0.13	0.89	0.18±0.41$^{\&}$ & P=0.02	-1.02	0.31
	Control Group（n=11）	0.88±0.84			0.50±0.76		
Diurnal variation	Feedback Group（n=13）	0.27±0.91	-0.16	0.88	0.27±0.65	-1.24	0.22
	Control Group（n=11）	0.13±0.35			0.00±0.00		
Block	Feedback Group（n=13）	6.27±1.49	-0.42	0.68	2.55±1.81$^{\&\&}$ && P=0.01	-2.10	0.04*
	Control Group（n=11）	5.50±2.73			4.25±1.58		
Desperation	Feedback Group（n=13）	4.64±1.69	-0.38	0.71	2.64±1.03$^{\&}$ & P=0.02	-0.68	0.50
	Control Group（n=11）	4.00±2.93			3.25±2.19		

Impacts on Anxiety. There were significant differences in the feedback group before and after treatment in Mental anxiety factor score (from 12.64±2.80 to 6.91±3.48, P=0.00), Somatic anxiety factor score (from 5.73±3.44 to 2.00±1.95, P=0.01) and the Total Score of HAMA (from 18.36±5.95to 8.91±5.01, P=0.00) in HAMA scale. Scores of the above factors all decreased after treatment. While no significant difference was found in the control group, as shown in Table 3.

There was no significant difference between the two groups in HAMA scale.

Table 3. Comparison of HAMA Factors and Total Score ($\overline{x} \pm s$, sum of ranks)

Item	Group	Baseline	F	Sig.	Follow-up	F	Sig.
Mental anxiety	Feedback Group（n=13）	12.64±2.80	0.73	0.40	6.91±3.48$^{\&\&}$ && P=0.00	0.96	0.34
	Control Group（n=11）	11.50±2.93			8.38±2.83		
Somatic anxiety	Feedback Group（n=13）	5.73±3.44	0.23	0.64	2.00±1.949$^{\&\&}$ && P=0.01	1.03	0.32
	Control Group（n=11）	5.00±3.02			3.25±3.41		
Total Scores	Feedback Group（n=13）	18.36±5.95	0.51	0.48	8.91±5.01$^{\&\&}$ && P=0.00	1.24	0.28
	Control Group（n=11）	16.50±5.04			11.63±5.55		

3.2   Impacts of HRV Biofeedback on Sleep

There were significant differences in the following components in the feedback group before and after treatment, that was, Sleep disturbance component score (from 1.55±1.29 to 0.55±0.82, P=0.03), Global PSQI Score (from 12.00±6.66 to 7.18±3.82, P=0.02), Subjective sleep quality component score (from 1.73±1.01 to 1.00±0.63, P=0.03), Sleep duration component score (from 1.64±1.36 to 0.45±0.93, P=0.03) and Daytime dysfunction component score (from 2.45±0.69 to 1.64±0.81, P=0.05). Scores of the above factors all decreased after treatment. The difference was not found in the control group, as shown in Table 4 and Table 5.

There was significant differences in the feedback group before and after treatment in Global PSQI Score (F=8.49, P=0.01), Subjective sleep quality component score (Z=-2.47, P=0.01) and Daytime dysfunction component score (Z=-2.35, P=0.02) after treatment, and scores of the feedback group were lower than that of the control group. The score of Sleep latency component of the feedback group was less than that of the other, with P close to 0.05(F=3.87, P=0.07), as shown in Table 4 and Table 5.

Table 4. Comparison of PQSI Components and Total Score ($\overline{x} \pm s$, t)

Item	Group	Baseline	F	Sig.	Follow-up	F	Sig.
Sleep duration	Feedback Group（n=13）	1.82±1.25	1.15	0.30	1.09±0.94	3.87	0.07
	Control Group（n=11）	2.38±0.92			2.13±1.36		
Sleep efficiency	Feedback Group（n=13）	1.55±1.29	0.08	0.78	0.55±0.82& & P=0.03	1.11	0.31
	Control Group（n=11）	1.38±1.30			1.00±1.07		
Global PSQI Score	Feedback Group（n=13）	12.00±6.66	0.24	0.63	7.18±3.82& & P=0.02	8.49	0.01**
	Control Group（n=11）	13.38±5.01			12.13±3.40		

Table 5. Comparison of PQSI Components and Total Score ($\overline{x} \pm s$, sum of ranks)

Item	Group	Baseline	Z	Sig.	Follow-up	Z	Sig.
Subjective sleep quality	Feedback Group（n=13）	1.73±1.01	-1.43	0.15	1.00±0.63& & P=0.03	-2.47	0.01*
	Control Group（n=11）	2.38±0.74			1.88±0.84		
Sleep duration	Feedback Group（n=13）	1.64±1.36	-0.04	0.97	0.45±0.93& & P=0.03	-1.63	0.10
	Control Group（n=11）	1.63±1.30			1.38±1.41		
Sleep disturbance	Feedback Group（n=13）	1.18±0.60	-0.93	0.35	1.00±0.45	-0.65	0.52
	Control Group（n=11）	1.00±0.00			1.13±0.35		
Daytime dysfunction	Feedback Group（n=13）	2.45±0.69	0.00	1.00	1.64±0.81& & P=0.05	-2.35	0.02*
	Control Group（n=11）	2.38±0.92			2.63±0.74		

3.3   Impacts of HRV Biofeedback on Motor Function, Damage Levels and Activities of Daily Living

There were significant differences in the feedback group before and after treatment in the total score of FMA scale (from 48.64±30.36 to 53.64±30.22, P=0.01), NIHSS scale (from 6.82±5.08 to 4.91±4.11, P=0.00) and MBI scale (from 55.91±23.86 to 67.27±19.66, P=0.0). The total score of FMA scale and MBI scale increased while those of NIHSS scale decreased. The control group also showed significant differences in the total score of FMA scale (from 24.75±10.57 to 32.38±11.35, P=0.00), NIHSS scale (from 10.25±1.67 to 8.00±1.93, P=0.00) and MBI scale (from 36.25±12.17 to 51.25±15.30, P=0.00) after treatment, with total scores of FMA and MBI scale increasing and those of NIHSS scale decreasing, as shown in Table 6.

There was no significant difference between the two groups in FMA, NIHSS and MBI scales, as shown in Table 6.

Table 6. Comparison of Total Score in FMA , NIHSS and MBI scales ($\overline{x} \pm s$, sum of ranks)

Item	Group	Baseline	Z	Sig.	Follow-up	Z	Sig.
Motor Function	Feedback Group (n=13)	48.64±30.36	-1.82	0.07	53.64±30.22[&] & P=0.01	-1.49	0.14
	Control Group (n=11)	24.75±10.57			32.38±11.35[&&] && P=0.00		
Stroke Scale	Feedback Group (n=13)	6.82±5.08	-1.08	0.28	4.91±4.11[&&] && P=0.00	-1.37	0.17
	Control Group (n=11)	10.25±1.67			8.00±1.93[&&] && P=0.00		
Barthel Index	Feedback Group (n=13)	55.91±23.86	-1.78	0.08	67.27±19.67[&&] && P=0.00	-1.62	0.11
	Control Group (n=11)	36.25±12.17			51.25±15.30[&&] && P=0.00		

3.4   Impacts of HRV Biofeedback on HRV Indices

Time-Domain Analysis. There was significant difference in the feedback and control group before and after treatment, as shown in Table 7.

Table 7. Comparison of HR and SDNN ($\overline{x} \pm s$, sum of ranks)

Item	Group	Baseline	F	Sig.	Follow-up	F	Sig.
Heart Rate (Beats / min)	Feedback Group (n=13)	80.20±9.46	0.07	0.80	79.97±14.28	0.61	0.45
	Control Group (n=11)	78.87±12.60			74.65±15.30		
SDNN (ms)	Feedback Group (n=13)	36.19±24.15	-0.50	0.62	44.62±32.23	-2.23	0.03[*]
	Control Group (n=11)	35.15±35.50			18.22±11.27		

There was no significant difference on SDNN after treatment (Z=-2.23, P=0.03 respectively), with scores of the feedback group apparently higher than those of the control group, as shown in Table 7.

Frequency-Domain Analysis. In the feedback group before and after treatment, the results were as follows: In the frequency domain analysis, there were significant differences on rank and test of LF(from 62.17±114.91 to 273.93±462.78, P=0.05) and LF/HF(from 0.97±0.70 to 8.52±16.66, P=0.03) of the feedback group, with scores increasing apparently. As shown in Table 8, the rank and test of the control group had no differences.

There was significant difference on LF after treatment (Z=-2.97, P=0.00 respectively), with scores of the feedback group apparently higher than those of the control group, as shown in Table 8.

Table 8. Comparison of LF, HF and LF/HF ($\overline{x} \pm s$, sum of ranks)

Item	Group	Baseline	Z	Sig.	Follow-up	Z	Sig.
LF (ms)	Feedback Group(n=13)	62.18±114.91	-0.50	0.62.	273.93±462.78$^{\&}$ $_{\& P=0.05}$	-2.97	0.00**
	Control Group(n=11)	77.69±147.72			16.36±25.63		
HF (ms)	Feedback Group(n=13)	71.31±84.77	-0.58	0.56	98.80±218.17	-1.32	0.19
	Control Group(n=11)	190.56±405.96			23.95±39.93		
LF/HF	Feedback Group(n=13)	0.97±0.70	-0.79	0.43	8.52±16.66$^{\&}$ $_{\& P=0.03}$	-1.32	0.19
	Control Group(n=11)	0.82±0.62			2.01±2.19		

3.5   Impacts of HRV Biofeedback on Respiratory

There was significant difference in the feedback group before and after treatment on respiratory rate(from 15.89±1.39 to 11.60±3.31, Unit: beats / min, P=0.00), with scores decreasing. While no difference in control group was found.

There was significant difference on respiratory rate after treatment (F=12.86, P=0.00), with scores of the feedback group apparently lower than those of the control group, as shown in Table 9.

Table 9. Comparison of Respiratory ($\overline{x} \pm s$, t)

Item	Group	Baseline	F	Sig.	Follow-up	F	Sig.
Resprate (br/min)	Feedback Group(n=13)	15.89±1.39	0.77	0.39	11.60±3.31$^{\&\&}$ $_{\&\& P=0.00}$	12.86	0.00*
	Control Group(n=11)	16.68±2.04			16.04±1.29		

4   Discussion

This study reveals that 10 times HRV biofeedback is an effective treatment for post-stroke depression patients with no side effects caused by the intervention of antidepressant drugs. According to the HRV data collected in our experiment, all patients who completed the training have mastered the method of carrying out HRV biofeedback, and can take the initiative to apply this breathing method to daily life. Results showed significant differences between the group taking HRV biofeedback treatment and the group breathing at resonance frequency (5.5 to 6 times per minute). One significant difference between the two groups was LF ($Z=-2.97$, $P=0.00$ respectively) after treatment, with the score of the feedback group apparently higher than that of the control group. This showed that the LF value of the feedback group was apparently higher than that of the control group after treatment (Table 8). The other significant difference was the respiratory rate ($F=12.86$, $P=0.00$), with the score of the feedback group apparently lower than that of the control group. This showed that the respiratory rate of the feedback group was apparently lower than that of the control group after treatment (Table 9). That is, respiratory rate decreased while volatility of LF increased significantly. As the most important index of HRV biofeedback, the more significantly LF increases the stronger patients' feedback awareness and ability as well as their regulation on autonomic function level. This finding is consistent with those of most experiments, that is, LF increases significantly in the feedback process [8-12]. Mechanism for the change of HRV is unclear at present. After lots of authoritative research, Lehrer thought that the increase of HRV was caused by stimulation of baroreflex [12-14]. And the baroreflex also plays an important role in achieving homeostatic state of autonomic function and the adaptability of entire cardiovascular system. Obviously, HRV biofeedback strengthens sinus arrhythmia and enhances its volatility and variability, and under certain conditions, there is a synchronous effect between such fluctuations and baroreflex [14-16]. Only when patients breathe at resonance frequency, baroreflex will be activated to the greatest extent. And its activity will be enhanced by constantly strengthening the feedback training. By behavioral therapy, patients strengthen the control of self-regulation on autonomic nervous function, which indicates the improvement of functional activity of vagus nerve [17].

Our experiment found that although the clinical symptoms, both the depressive symptoms and the anxiety symptoms, were obviously changed, unlike the Karavidas [9] results in significant improvement, the depression and anxiety levels and the mild depression and anxiety levels still didn't reach the clinical cure levels after 10 times' treatment. Is this because patients with post-stroke depression are not more sensitive to HRV biofeedback? Or is this because the process of feedback treatment for patients with post-stroke depression is different from that for patients with other diseases? I think the disease specificity of post-stroke depression disease may account for this. The pathogenesis of PSD is complex, and is currently thought to be related to various factors. There is no unified point of view, and it's considered to be a result of both neurobiological and psychosocial factors. Most scholars favor the theory of "biological mechanism", which believes that the parts of the brain damaged and neurotransmitters are important factors in determining whether stroke patients suffer from depression. In addition, many studies have found that, cytokines can excessively activate the hypothalamic-pituitary-adrenal axis (HPA axis), and cause damage to the receptor function of glucocorticoid [18]. And thus it will decrease its response to corticosteroids, leading to no inhibition of the inflammatory response, the rise of plasma cortisol, corticotrophin releasing hormone (CRH) and adrenocorticotropic hormone (ACTH) levels, and the hyperactivity of sympathetic nervous system which then causes corresponding behaviors and emotional changes [18]. The release of hormones, as well as breaking the balance function of autonomic, sympathetic and vagal nerves, is closely related to HRV-related indicators. Although the observed indicators of the study did not involve the measure of various neurotransmitter and hormone levels, previous studies have showed that the anxiety and depression combined stroke has a greater impact on HRV than mere stroke or simply depression, and its damage on autonomic nerve is more serious. We can guess that, due to the special nature of the pathogenesis of post-stroke depression, as well as the occurrence and evolution distinguished from other types of depression, the efficacy of HRV biofeedback on stroke depression is different from previous experimental results. Based on the above results, our experiment found that after 10 times HRV biofeedback, depression and anxiety levels of patients were still in the recovery process, but they were not completely cured. There exists a need to increase the frequency and intensity of training to observe its long-term effect. The recovery mechanism of HRV biofeedback therapy for stroke patients with depression needs to be further studied.

The study also found that although motor function, disability level and activities of daily living were improved significantly when depression consistently changed with HRV indices, there was no apparent difference between the two groups. See Table 11. Although the occurrence of depression after stroke has a close relationship to patients' paralyze, the reduce in their capacity for activities of daily living and their inability to take care of themselves, studies have also found that their relationship is non-synchronous. Next step, we'll extend the follow-up time, add observed indicators of prognosis, and clarify their level of efficacy.

The experiment has also found that HRV biofeedback can significantly improve sleep disturbance of stroke patients with depression, which is a bright spot of our results. Between the two groups, there were significant differences on Sleep disturbance factor of HAMD (F=7.88, P=0.01), Subjective sleep quality component of PQSI (Z = -2.47, P = 0.01), Daytime dysfunction component (Z=-2.35, P=0.02) and Global PSQI Score (F=8.50, P=0.01). The fact that scores of the feedback group were apparently lower than those of the control group indicated the improvement of sleep quality, daytime functional status and overall sleep of feedback group after treatment. Sleep latency component of PQSI is close to 0.05 (F=3.87, P=0.07) after treatment. Sleep latency component of the feedback group was apparently lower than that of the control group, showing that there was a downward trend in sleep latency after treatment, yet it was not statistically significant compared to the control group (Table1, Table4-5). HRV biofeedback promote a conversion of autonomic nervous activity to be conducive to sleep and also a decline in awakened level, which will then induce sleep[19], increase depth of sleep, improve sleep quality and shorten sleep latency. Our experiment also found that patients felt significant improvements of their daytime function. This may be due to shorter sleep time and an overall improvement of sleep quality, so that patients get adequate rest and are able to energetically engage in various rehabilitation activities in the daytime, which is of great clinical value in the improvement of neurological deficit and activities of daily living for stroke patients.

5   Conclusion and Future Work

We applied Heart Rate Variability (HRV) biofeedback to train PSD patients by a prospective randomized control study. This study reveals effectiveness of the HRV biofeedback on stroke patients' emotional improvement, autonomic nerve function and prognostic implications. HRV biofeedback is a beneficial adjuvant treatment for patients with post-stroke depression in rehabilitation training. Our findings suggest that 10 times HRV biofeedback is an effective treatment for post-stroke depression patients, especially on the improvement of depression levels and sleep disturbance.

The theory for the long-term effect of LF (i.e., the follow-up efficacy some time after HRV biofeedback) is unclear so far. Our experiment has found that after 10 times HRV biofeedback, depression and anxiety levels of patients are still higher than normal and there was no significant difference on the improvement of motor function, disability level and activities of daily living between two groups. In the next treatment design, we need to increase the frequency or intensity of training, or extend the long-term follow-up time to 2-3 months or longer, so as to study the long-term effect and mechanisms of HRV biofeedback for stroke patients with depression.

Acknowledgements. This study was supported by the National Basic Research Program of China (973 Program) No.2011CB302302. We would like to thank Dechun Sang, Songhuai Liu, Lin Wang, Shufeng Ji, from Bo Ai Hospital, Beijing. We also appreciate the research assistance provided by Yan Zhang MSc from Tsinghua University.

References

1. Ming-ming, Y.: Relationship among Depression, Anxiety and Possible Factors in Post-stroke Patients: 510 Cases Report. Chinese Journal of Rehabilitation Theory and Practice 12(6), 498–500 (2006)
2. Dai-qun, X., Rong, Y., Rong-mei, L., et al.: Analysis of Post-stroke Anxiety Disorders and the Related Factors. Huaxi Medicine 19(1), 133 (2004)
3. Karavidas, M.K., Lehrer, P.M., Vaschillo, E.G., Vaschillo, B., Humberton, M., Buyske, S., et al.: Preliminary results of an open label study of heart rate variability biofeedback for the treatment of major depression. Applied Psychophysiology and Biofeedback 32, 19–30 (2007)

4. Zucker, T.L., Samuelson, K.W., Muench, F., Greenberg, M.A., Gevirtz, R.N.: The effects of respiratory sinus arrhythmia biofeedback on heart rate variability and posttraumatic stress disorder symptoms, A pilot study. Applied Psychophysiology & Biofeedback 34, 135–143 (2009)
5. National Conference on Cerebrovascular Disease Score Standards in Clinical Neurological Deficit for Stroke Patients. Chinese Journal of Neurology 29(6), 381–383 (1995)
6. World Health Organization. ICD-10:The ICD-10 Classification of Mental and Behavioural Disorders: Clinical Descriptions and Diagnostic Guidelines, Geneva (1992)
7. Randomized Controlled Trials Table, http://www.randomizer.org/form.htm
8. Hassett, A.L., Radvanski, D.C., Vaschillo, E.G., et al.: A pilot study of the efficacy of heart rate variability (HRV) biofeedback in patients with fibromyalgia. Applied Psychophysiology and Biofeedback 32, 1–10 (2007)
9. Karavidas, M.K., Leherer, P.M., Vaschillo, E., et al.: Preliminary results of an open lable study of heart rate variability biofeedback for the treatment of major depression. Applied Psychophysiology and Biofeedback 32, 19–30 (2007)
10. Lehrer, P., Carr, R., Smetankine, A., Vaschillo, E., Peper, E., Porges, S., et al.: Respiratory sinus arrhythmia versus neck/ trapezius EMG and incentive inspirometry biofeedback for asthma, A pilot study. Applied Psychophysiology & Biofeedback 22, 95–109 (1997)
11. Lehrer, P., Vaschillo, E., Vaschillo, B., Lu, S., Eckberg, D., Edelberg, R., et al.: Heart rate variability biofeedback increases baroreflex gain and peak expiratory flow. Psychosomatic Medicine 65, 796–805 (2003)
12. Lehrer, P., Vaschillo, E., Vaschillo, B., Lu, S., Scardella, A., Siddique, M., et al.: Biofeedback treatment for asthma. Chest. 126, 352–361 (2004)
13. Lehrer, P., Vaschillo, E., Lu, S., Eckberg, D., Vaschillo, B., Scardella, A., et al.: Heart rate variability biofeedback, Effects of age on heart rate variability, baroreflex gain, and asthma. Chest. 129, 278–284 (2006)
14. Lehrer, P.M.: Applied psychophysiology, Beyond the boundaries of biofeedback (mending a wall, a brief history of our field, and applications to control of the muscles and cardiorespiratory systems). Applied Psychophysiology and Biofeedback 28(4), 291–304 (2003)
15. Vaschillo, E.G., Lehrer, P.M., Rishe, N., Konstantinov, M.: Heart rate variability biofeedback as a method for assessing baroreflex function, A preliminary study of resonance in the cardiovascular system. Applied Psychophysiology and Biofeedback 27(1), 1–27 (2002)
16. Maria, K.K., Paul, M.L., Evgeny, V., et al.: Preliminary Results of an Open Label Study of Heart RateVariability Biofeedback for the Treatment of Major Depression. Appl. Psychophysiol Biofeedback 32, 19–30 (2007)
17. Vaschillo, E.G., Vaschillo, B., Lehrer, P.M.: Characteristics of resonance in heart rate variability stimulated by biofeedback. Applied Psychophysiology and Biofeedback 31(2), 129–142 (2006)
18. Pawate, S., Shen, Q., Fan, F., et al.: Redox regulation of glial inflammatory response to lipopolysaccharide and interfere on gamma. J. Neurosci. Res. 77(4), 540–551 (2004)
19. Ya-lin, Z.: Behavior Therapy. Guizhou People's Publishing House, Guiyang (1990)

Optimal ST-Elevation Myocardial Infarction System by Regional Cooperative Emergency Care Based on the Internet of Things

Hao Chen[1,4], Dingcheng Xiang[1], Weiyi Qin[1], Minwei Zhou[1], Ji-Jiang Yang[2], Qiang Gao[3], and Jian Liu[1]

[1] Guangzhou General Hospital of Guangzhou Military Command, Guangzhou, China, 510010
13889903869@139.com
[2] RIIT, Tsinghua University, Beijing, China, 100084
yangjijiang@tsinghua.edu.cn
[3] IVT (Beijing) Technology Inc., Beijing, China, 100085
[4] HuaBo BioPharmaceutical Institute of GuangZhou, Guangzhou, China, 510010

Abstract. Prompt reperfusion treatment significantly reduces mortality and morbidity in patients with ST-elevation myocardial infarction (STEMI). In this article, the current status and problems of STEMI patient emergency care were studied and key influence factors were found. A regional cooperative emergency care system for STEMI patients were established based on the internet of things. An expedited pre-hospital diagnosis and transfer pathway was developed, as a result of which, a shorter time from symptom onset to reperfusion was achieved and the outcome for patients was improved.

Keywords: internet of things, ST-segment elevation myocardial infarction, mhealth system, primary percutaneous coronary intervention.

1 Introduction

The internet of things is a network that uses radio frequency identification (RFID), infrared sensors, global positioning system, laser scanners and other sensing devices to connect any object to the Internet for information exchange and communication by agreed protocols so as to realize intelligent identification, positioning, tracking, monitoring and management [1]. The internet of things, as an emerging information technique, is gradually introduced into the medical industry [2]. How to create an emergency care network system for ST-segment elevation myocardial infarction (STEMI) by adopting internet of things as well as optimizing the process of emergency medical services (EMS), so as to effectively integrate the pre-hospital and in-hospital rescue and shorten the diagnosis and treatment time for STEMI patients, is a valuable topic worth of study.

Acute STEMI is usually caused by complete obstruction of coronary artery when the atherosclerotic plaque in coronary artery ruptures and the platelets and coagulation process is activated [3]. Large number of evidence-based medical researches show that

X. Zheng et al. (Eds.): ICSH 2014, LNCS 8549, pp. 225–232, 2014.
© Springer International Publishing Switzerland 2014

the shorter the infarct-related artery is obstructed, the greater the possibility the patient is likely to be rescued, and that the occlusion time of the infarct-related artery is a key factor that would influence the infarct size and prognosis of patients. The American college of cardiology (ACC)/American heart association (AHA) guideline recommended that the ideal time window of reperfusion is within 2 hours after the onset of acute myocardial infarction, and that the door-to-balloon (D2B) time is < 90 min, which is also used as a quality control standard [5]. The onset-to-treatment and D2B time is crucial to the chain of survival for the STEMI patients, the reduction of which would save more heart and brain function and hence reduce the disability and mortality rates. With this purpose, several domestic hospitals specially create Green Channels to simplify the process of the diagnosis and treatment of STEMI, but find the results not so satisfactory. The main reason is that the emergency care process of STEMI consists of the pre-hospital and in-hospital treatment, and only optimizing and effectively managing the whole process will lead to a real reduction of time for emergency care. Therefore, to provide basis for the optimization of process, it is necessary to analyze the key links and influential factors from the onset of STEMI to the diagnosis and treatment of the disease.

It is a continuous process from the onset of STEMI to reperfusion, and the delay of treatment mainly includes pre-hospital delay and in-hospital delay. The pre-hospital delay usually occurs before the patients ask for emergency medical help and during the emergency transport, and the in-hospital delay usually occurs during the process of examination, triage, medical consultation, and the definitive treatment. Considering that the time delay is a main reason leading to the failure of treatment, an analysis of the distribution and influential factors of the delay may provide strategic support for the optimization of the emergency process, including, how to transport patients from hospitals without interventional capabilities to capable hospitals, and how to optimize the internal process of the latter [6-8].

Currently, reperfusion therapy mainly includes the thrombolytic drug therapy and percutaneous coronary intervention therapy (PCI), in which PCI is preferred, because after STEMI patients received thrombolytic therapy, regardless of the success, they would benefit the most from PCI treatment within 3 to 24 hours. However, since our country has vast expanse of land and large population, and the current health care resources are unevenly distributed, the patients' onset-to-treatment time is varied and the delay for medical help is common. Meanwhile, considering the catheterization labs and the qualifications of physicians, many patients were sent to hospitals without PCI capabilities and hence cannot get the maximum benefit from PCI. Even in some developed Euro-American countries with the best medical transport systems, there are long delays for the transfer of patients with chest pain, especially in rural or mountain areas. It cannot be achieved in a short time to meet the conditions of time, place and emergency medical staff for instant PCI. Therefore, as the evidence-based medicine requires, the best PCI treatment program has to be selected based on the clinical practice (including the willingness of patients and the medical skills of rescue staff) [9]. Nowadays, many guidelines propose that, PCI therapy should be implemented directly after the onset of STEMI and the time between the first treatment and the D2B shall be less than 90min [10].

2   System Design

Taking chest pain center as an opportunity, a military hospital adopted the internet of things, remote medical services, mobile medical services and other information techniques into the construction and created the first chest pain emergency network system based on internet of things in the world [11,12]. In the emergency process management of STEMI patients, modern information technology was integrated with process management, so that the emergency process management extended from in-hospital to pre-hospital and transport process. Through monitoring and real-time guidance to the whole process of emergency care, it was possible to manage time and mobility of medical behavior so as to realize a seamless connection of different sections of medical treatment for STEMI patients. Also, the hospital made full use of its good organization and coordination as a large military 3A hospital, its pre-hospital emergency brand and advanced catheterization techniques, the resources of military and civilian joint hospitals, community hospitals and large business units to achieve the multi-disciplinary (including pre-hospital EMS, emergency department, cardiology department, imaging department) cooperation and multi-level hospitals (community hospitals, fundamental hospitals, central hospital) linkage. In this way, with the specialists from large hospitals as core strength, secondary hospitals as key strength and the community and family as the supporting level, a STEMI emergency network system was established, which provided medical services with shared information, institution network, advanced specialists and helpful personnel [13].

The STEMI emergency network system is established based on the structure of "information collection, data transmission and data processing" and adopts the technology of the internet of things. With the help of these technologies, the data of vital signs including 12-lead electrocardiogram (ECG), blood pressure, oxygen saturation, blood glucose of the patients' at the network hospitals, emergency stations, or in the ambulances are transmitted timely to the chest pain center through 3G network or satellite channels as shown in Fig. 1. In this way, the cardiologists from chest pain center or physicians on duty of cardiology department can remotely monitor the status for diagnosis and treatment. As for those patients who need to be transferred to the general hospital for emergency treatment, they will be directly sent to the Coronary Care Unit (CCU) of the general hospital by the ambulances. As for the patients with acute myocardial infarction (AMI) who need emergency interventional treatment, preparation of the catheterization lab and the preoperative preparation shall start when the patients are still in the ambulance, so that they would be directly sent to the catheterization lab upon their arrival. Since the emergency department is bypassed and the preoperative preparation is done in the ambulance on the way to the target hospital, it significantly shortens the patients' time window from onset to operation, which saves precious time for emergency treatment, especially for the acute STEMI patients who need immediate PCI therapy.

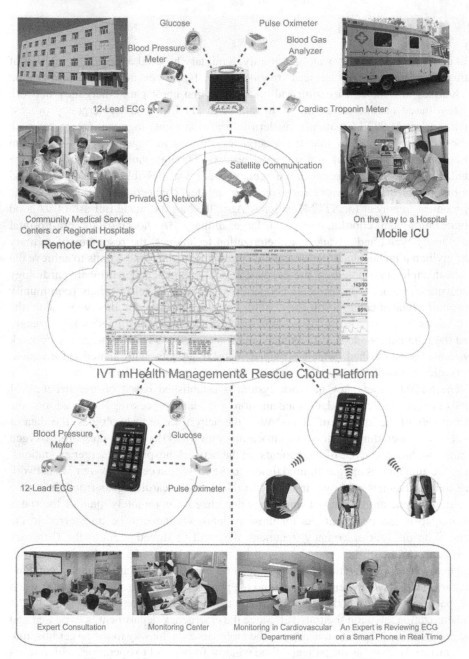

Fig. 1. Architecture of mHealth System Using Internet of Things

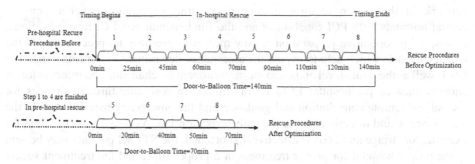

1.12-Lead ECG in ER; 2.Specialist Consultation; 3.Notify the Operation Staff; 4.Doctors Arrive at the Catheterization Laboratory;5.Check/Supplement All the Materials;6.Operation Preparations;7.An Operation Get Started;8.Balloon-opening is done

Fig. 2. The emergency process before and after the STEMI emergency network system was established

3   Outcome

Since the STEMI emergency network system was established on March 27, 2011, a total of 754 patients with chest pain had been rescued during one-year operation (i.e. April 1, 2011 to March 30, 2012), and the treatment success ratio was 97.5%. Among the cases, the median D2B time of STEMI patients is 69 min, of which the shortest time is 21 min, and 82.5% was less than 90 min, better than the international standard[5] (median D2B time is 90 min, and no less than 75% is below 90 min).

4   Discussion

The World Health Organization (WHO) statistics show that every year, many patients died of myocardial infarction at home or on the site in the first few hours from onset, for they have failed to be sent timely to the hospital. The most important delay factor for treatment is the pre-hospital delay, which accounts for 75% of the delay time and mostly due to the delay of the patients themselves. Hence, the solution for pre-hospital delay lies in promoting and popularizing the emergency knowledge and skills of the public, encouraging the patients to "speed to hospital when chest pain occurs", conducting comprehensive risk analysis for cardiovascular patients and establishing the mechanisms of prediction, prevention, early warning and plans for patients. Besides, the delay of transport is mainly affected in three stages--the hospital the patients first turn to, the transport process and the hospital that receives the patients, and in our country, the pre-hospital delay mainly happens in the first two stages [14]. With the help of "remote intensive care unit (ICU)" and "Mobile ICU", if the patients cannot be transferred for immediate PCI therapy within 90 min, they would first receive thrombolytic therapy in the network hospitals, and later be transferred to central hospital for PCI therapy, which is an effective way to improve the fist diagnosis, shorten the pre-hospital delay so as to ensure the safety of the patients. Furthermore, according to the regional health planning of China, an effective STEMI emergency network in the region requires a cooperative transfer relationship between the central hospitals with PCI capabilities and the fundamental non-PCI hospitals. Some in-hospital preoperative preparation is now moved to pre-hospital process due to the Green Channels which help to bypass the emergency department to the catheterization lab as well as the multi-level and cooperative treatment mechanism. The information of patients such as pre-hospital ECG is transmitted in real time through devices for specialists' remote consultation and guidance and the emergency medical staff in the ambulance would directly activate the catheterization lab. As a result, as the time for examination, triage and D2B is effectively shortened, the STEMI patients may be sent to the proper hospital for proper treatment in a proper time, and the treatment sucess ratio is therefore raised [15, 16]. Domestic study also reported that pre-hospital ECG can significantly shorten the D2B time of STEMI patients, but the study still needs further improvement due to the fact that the pre-hospital ECG completion rate is low[17].

Given that the in-hospital delay accounts for only 1/4 of the total delay time and it is highly controllable, it is another key factor to shorten the overall delay time. How to reduce the D2B time has become an important index for improving the treatment sucess of STEMI patients that received immediate PCI therapy. According to the guideline, the recommended D2B time is 90 min, with 75% D2B time less than 90 min [5]. However, according to the domestic and international clinical practice, especially for the domestic practice, there is still a way to achieve the requirements of the guideline. In developed Euro-American countries, the median D2B time is 55min ~ 147min, only less than 15% hospitals is lower than 90 min and the D2B is 4.2%~80% of the target value of the guideline[5,18-21]. Domestic study reported that the median D2B time was 92min~135min, only 18.1% ~58.4% reached the target value of D2B of the guideline [17, 22-27].

The establishment of effective cooperative mechanism and emergency medical teams among hospitals would significantly reduce the D2B time. In this study, a 24/7 interventional team was provided. Before the arrival of STEMI patients, the treatment plan was initiated--the catheterization lab would be prepared and all medical staff was ready within 30 min--to make sure the STEMI patients received treatment in the shortest time.

The D2B time can be significantly shortened by means of PH-ECG and bypassing the Emergency Department to directly enter the catheterization lab. The early diagnosis of ECG is made by experienced cardiovascular specialist so as to reduce the false positive rate. Also, guidance shall be provided to the medical staff of pre-hospital emergency, which, however, is based on the high quality information collection. The collection rate of pre-hospital ECG of STEMI patients was not satisfactory and the completion rate was 36%, most of which was collected through EMS [17]. It shows that there is an urgent need to increase popularity of related knowledge among the public, to train more public emergency physicians and to increase the number of emergency centers.

5   Conclusion

In conclusion, in accordance with the relevant professional guideline for STEMI treatment, a regional cooperative emergency network based on the internet of things was created, which contains the linkage of emergency factors, the linkage of time and process as well as the linkage of spatial distribution. The technology of internet of things was integrated to the process management of STEMI emergency, and the specific rescue process and application was integrated to the operation of network. As a result, the process from the onset to pre-hospital emergency to in-hospital emergency has been optimized and simplified, the onset-to-reperfusion time has been shortened and the treatment success rate has been raised.

Acknowledgments. Sponsored by the PhD Start-up Fund of Natural Science Foundation of Guangdong Province, China, S2013040012611; Science and Technology Program of Guangdong Province, China, 2010B031500015.

References

1. Gong, L.D.R., Shao, J.R.: From digital earth to intelligence earth. Wuhan University Journal 35(2), 127–132 (2010)
2. Chen, H., Li, S.Z., Chen, L.M., et al.: Construction and application of remote medical health monitoring platform based on body area network. Chinese Journal of Social Medicine 28(5), 300–302 (2011)
3. Libby, P.: Current concepts of the pathogenesis of the acute coronary syndromes. Circulation 104(3), 365–372 (2001)
4. Henry, T.D., Unger, B.T., Sharkley, S.W., et al.: Design of standardized system for transfer of patients with ST-elevation myocardial infarction for percutaneous coronary intervention. Am. Heart J. 150(3), 373–384 (2005)
5. Antman, E.M., Hand, M., Amstrong, P.W., et al.: Focused Up-date of the ACC/AHA 2004 Guidelines for the Management of Patients with St-Elevation Myocardial Infarction: A report of the American College of Cardiology/American Heart Association Task Force on Practice Guidelines. Circulation 117, 296–329 (2008)
6. Wang, J., Guo, J.C.: A Survey on Pre-hospital Delay of Acute ST-elevation Myocardial Infarction Patients. Practical Journal of Cardiac Cerebral Pneumal and Vascular Disease 17(8), 651–652 (2009)
7. Song, L., Yan, H.B., Yang, J.G., et al.: A Study on Influence of Different Clinical Paths to Door-to-Balloon Time of Acute ST-elevation Myocardial Infarction Patients. Practical Journal of Cardiac Cerebral Pneumal and Vascular Disease 30(2), 99–102 (2011)
8. Zhang, Q., Shen, W.F.: A Strategy of Transferred PCI Therapy for Acute ST-elevation Myocardial Infarction. International Journal of Cardiovascular Disease 36(6), 328–332 (2009)
9. Liu, Y.X., Li, W.M.: A Discussion on Interventional Therapy of ST-elevation Myocardial Infarction of Reperfusion Guideline. International Journal of Cardiovascular Disease 38(1), 14–17 (2011)
10. The Task Force on Myocardial Revascularization of the European Society of Cardiology (ESC) and the European Association for Cardio-Thoracic Surgery(EACTS).Guidelines on myocardial revascularization. Eur. J. Cardiothorac. Surg. 38(suppl), S1-S52 (2010)

11. Zhou, W.M.: Successful operation of the first military and civilian joint remote emergency internet of things in China. China Hospital CEO 19, 84–85 (2011)
12. Chen, H.: The operation of Chest Pain Emergency Network of Guangzhou General Hospital. e-Healthcare 5, 24 (2011)
13. Li, R., Zhang, L.: A study on continuous medical service model between hospitals and community-based health care stations. Medicine and Society 24(5), 55–57 (2011)
14. Zhang, Q., Zhang, R.Y., Qiu, J.P., et al.: Prospective multi-center randomized trial comparing physician versus patient transfer for primary percutaneous coronary intervention in acute ST-segment elevation myocardial infarction. Chin. Med. J. 121(6), 485–491 (2008)
15. Boden, W.E., Eagle, K., Granger, C.: Reperfusion strategies in acute ST-segment elevation myocardial infarction: A comprehensive review of contemporary management options. J. Am. Coll. Cardiology. 50(10), 917–929 (2007)
16. Jneid, H., Fonarow, G.C., Cannon, C.P., et al.: Impact of time of presentation on the care and outcomes of acute myocardial infarction. Circulation 117(9), 2502–2509 (2008)
17. Cheng, S.J., Yan, H.B., Wang, J., et al.: How pre-hospital ECG influence the Door-to-Balloon time of ST-elevation myocardial infarction patients. Journal of Third Military Medical University 31(12), 1222–1224 (2009)
18. McNamara, R.I., Herrin, J., Bradley, E.H., et al.: Hospital improvement in time to reperfusion in patients with acute myocardial infarction, 1999 to 2002. J. Am. Coll. Cardiol. 47, 45–51 (2006)
19. Nallamothu, B.K., Bates, E.R., Herrin, J., et al.: Times to treatment in transfer patients undergoing primary percutaneous coronary intervention in the United States: National Registry of Myocardial Infarction(NRMI)-3/4 analysis. Circulation 111(6), 761–767 (2005)
20. Khot, U.N., Johnson, M., et al Ramsey, C.: Emergency department physician activation of the catheterization laboratory and immediate transfer to an immediately available catheterization laboratory reduce door-to-balloon time in ST-elevation myocardial infarction. Circulation 116(1), 67–76 (2007)
21. Amit, G., Cafri, C., Gilutz, H., et al.: Benefit of direct ambulance to coronary care unit admission of acute myocardial infarction patients undergoing primary percutaneous intervention[J]. Int. J. Cardiol. 119(3), 355–358 (2007)
22. Guo, J.C., Ma, C.S., Xu, M., et al.: The door-to-balloon time and its influence to interventional emergency of acute ST-elevation myocardial infarction patients. Chinese Journal of Interventional Cardiology 18(1), 21–24 (2010)
23. Zhao, W., Guo, L.J.: The status of Door-to-Balloon time of ST-elevation myocardial infarction patients and the influencing factors. Chinese Journal of Internal Medicine 47, 727–730 (2008)
24. Qiu, J.P., Zhang, Q., Lu, J.D., et al.: Direct ambulance transport to catheterization laboratory reduces door-to-balloon time in patients with acute ST-segment elevation myocardial infarction undergoing primary percutaneous coronary intervention:the DIRCT-STEMI study. Chin. Med. J.(Engl.) 124(6), 805–810 (2011)
25. Cheng, S.J., Yan, H.B.: The influence of pre-hospital phone calls to the Door-to-Balloon time of middle aged ST-elevation myocardial infarction patients. Chinese Journal of Geriatrics 28, 453–456 (2009)
26. Song, L., Hu, D.Y., Yan, H.B., et al.: Influence of ambulance use on early reperfusion therapies for acute myocardial infarction. Chin. Med. J. (Engl.) 121, 771–775 (2008)
27. Yu, L.T., Zhu, J., Mister, R., et al.: A study on the registration of reperfusion therapy for acute ST-elevation coronary syndrome in some domestic hospitals. Chinese Journal of Cardiology 34, 593–597 (2006)

Author Index